Drugs in Sport:
The pressure
to perform

Drugs in Sport:
The pressure
to perform

British Medical Association

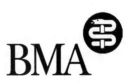

First published in 2002
by BMJ Books, BMA House, Tavistock Square,
London, WC1H 9JR

British Library Cataloguing in Publication Data

A catalogue record for this book is available from the British Library

ISBN 0 7279 1606 8

The photograph on the front cover is reproduced courtesy of PB Group Ltd.
Typeset by Saxon Graphics Ltd, Derby
Printed and bound in Spain by Graphycems, Navarra

Contents

Editorial Board

Board of Science and Education

This report was prepared under the auspices of the Board of Science and Education of the British Medical Association, whose membership for 2001/02 was as follows:

Acknowledgements

The Association is very grateful for the help provided by the BMA Committees and many outside experts and organisations and would particularly like to thank Dr Tim Crabbe, Dr Robert Dawson, and the Anti-Doping Directorate at UK Sport.

Approval for publication as a BMA policy report was recommended by BMA Executive Committee of Council on 14 November 2001.

1: Introduction

Background

The British Medical Association (BMA) is a professional organisation representing the medical profession in the UK. It was established in 1832 "to promote the medical and allied sciences, and to maintain the honour and interests of the profession". The Board of Science and Education, a standing committee of the Association, supports this aim by acting as an interface between the profession, the government and the public. Its main purpose is to contribute to the improvement of public health, and it has developed policies on a wide range of issues, including alcohol, the misuse of drugs, the therapeutic uses of cannabis, and sport and exercise medicine.

At various times throughout the 20th century drug misuse has concerned politicians, doctors and the public to varying degrees, and this has continued into the 21st century. Historically the attention devoted to drug misuse has not always related directly to the size or severity of the problem, but concern shown at today's drug use coincides with the real increase in overall levels of drug-taking observed since the late 1970s, particularly among young people. In addition, patterns of drug use have changed: there has been an increase in poly-drug use, including the combined use of licit and illicit drugs. The arrival of the "rave" scene has seen a resurgence in the use of LSD and amphetamines, and the introduction of new "dance drugs" such as ecstasy forms part of an increase in recreational and experimental drug use in the new millennium. However, the reasons for the use of drugs in sport and the problems caused by their misuse differ from those of recreational drugs, in that athletes take drugs in order to improve their athletic performance rather than as an end in itself.[1]

The BMA publication *Sport and exercise medicine: Policy and provision*[2] marked the establishment of BMA policy in relation to sports medicine. The aim of the report was to raise the profile of sports medicine and to assist those doctors with an interest in it. It concluded, among other things, that sporting bodies need to ensure they obtain medical advice in establishing rules and regulations that minimise the risk of injury to sports people, and that seeking medical advice in the area of drug use and abuse in sport is vital.

At the 2000 Annual Representative Meeting of the BMA it was resolved "That the BMA develop, through the Board of Science and Education, a policy on the use of performance-enhancing drugs in sport". This present study extends the BMA's policy on drugs and on sport into new areas to address this challenging resolution.

What is doping?

The International Olympic Committee (IOC) defines doping as "the use of an expedient (substance or method) which is potentially harmful to athletes' health and capable of enhancing their performance, or the presence in the athlete's body of a prohibited substance or evidence of the use thereof, or evidence of the use of a prohibited method".[3]

A universally accepted definition of a "performance-enhancing" drug remains elusive.

The term may be potentially misleading or restrictive in scope. Sports people may use drugs for a number of reasons other than for performance enhancement, including for legitimate therapeutic use, performance continuation, or recreational/social use. Those who fail drugs tests may not have intended to cheat. Hence, the IOC list of banned substances and methods includes prohibited substances and methods that may be taken or used by the athlete to enhance, maintain, or restore performance.

Whether a drug is considered to enhance performance depends on the context in which it is used. For example, β blockers may enhance performance in rifle shooting, but may well be dangerous or counter-productive if taken in another sport.[4] In addition, there is variability in the effects of drugs used by athletes. One research paper on three categories of drugs found a large individual variation in response to particular drugs. Many "performance-enhancing" drugs were found not to be as performance-enhancing as athletes supposed, and in certain circumstances were found actually to hinder performance.[5]

In an attempt to avoid using substances on the IOC banned list, sports people may use herbal remedies, sports supplements, and vitamins. These too must be considered as areas of "drugs in sport". The possible future use of biotechnology to enhance individuals genetically may complicate the terminology of "drugs" and "doping" in current usage.[6] Therefore, this report will explore the wider issue of drug use in sport and consider banned substances in general, not just those whose purpose is to enhance performance.

In summary, to define doping it may be useful to return to the definition provided by Sir Arthur Porrit, first chairman of the IOC Medical Commission: "To define doping is, if not impossible, at best extremely difficult, and yet everyone who takes part in competitive sport or who administers it knows exactly what it means. The definition lies not in words but in the integrity of the character" (quoted in Verroken[4]).

Aim and scope of the report

The purpose of this report is to provide information to doctors on what they may and may not prescribe to sports people, and the medical consequences of the use of certain drugs. It also intends to raise awareness of the medical and ethical issues surrounding the use of drugs in sports.

Following this introduction, Chapter 2 gives a brief overview of the historical, legal and ethical background to the subject, and Chapter 3 discusses the International Olympic Committee's list of banned substances and methods. This chapter provides an overview of each of the major classes of drugs, their potential use in sport, pharmacological actions, and adverse effects. It also considers therapeutic drugs used in the management of common illnesses. Chapter 4 details the use of anabolic androgenic steroids in British gymnasiums by non-competitive groups.

Chapter 5 considers the extent of doping in elite-level sports and some reasons for the apparent increase in drug use. Chapter 6 addresses the difficulty of reaching a consensus on the extent of the problem, the objectives of an anti-doping policy, and ways of tackling the problem. Chapter 7 looks at the role and responsibilities of doctors in doping in sport and the issues it raises for the medical profession. The final chapter draws conclusions and presents BMA recommendations for key actions by government, sporting organisations, health professionals, and a range of other interested parties.

The report and its recommendations should be of interest to doctors and other healthcare professionals, as well as those undertaking sporting activities, or providing training and coaching. It is intended that the recommendations will influence government to release additional resources to better enable the sporting community to tackle the major challenge of doping in sport.

References

1 Korkia PK, Stimson GV. *Anabolic steroid use in Great Britain: an exploratory investigation.* The Centre for Research on Drugs and Health Behaviour. A report for the Department of Health, the Welsh Office and the Chief Scientist Office, Scottish Home and Health Department, 1993.
2 British Medical Association. *Sport and exercise medicine: policy and provision.* London: BMA, 1996.
3 International Olympic Committee Medical Commission. *Olympic movement anti-doping code.* IOC, 1999.
4 Verroken M. Drug use and abuse in sport. In: DR Mottram, ed. *Drugs and sport:* 2nd edn. London: E&FN Spon, 1996.
5 Clarkson PM, Thompson HS. Drugs and sport: research findings and limitations. *Sports Medicine* 1997;**24**: 366–84.
6 Wadler GI. *Doping in sport: from strychnine to genetic enhancement, it's a moving target.* Duke Conference, 1999.

2: Setting the scene

History

There is a perception by some that doping in sport is a new phenomenon, and that there was once a time when sporting ethics prevailed. However, evidence of the use of various products to give athletes an advantage over their opponents can be traced back to the ancient Greeks in the third century BC, the ancient Egyptians and the Romans. Substances were derived from plants, including ginseng root, hemp, kava, opium, and hallucinogenic mushrooms, and from animals, such as steroids from sheep's testicles. In the 19th century caffeine, alcohol, ether, oxygen, cocaine, heroin, morphine, and strychnine were reported to have been used.[1] The first death suspected of being caused by doping in sport occurred in 1886, after a racing cyclist finished the Bordeaux–Paris race.[2]

Drugs were widely used by sportsmen and women in the 20th century. During the 1930s caffeine, alcohol, nitroglycerine, digitalis, cocaine, ether, opium, and heroin were drugs of choice.[2] Amphetamines were first used in the Berlin Olympics in 1936, and were heavily used until the 1970s. They were implicated in the deaths of three cyclists in 1960, 1967 and 1968. Anabolic steroids made their entry into sport in the 1940s and 1950s. The widespread use of sophisticated chemical agents began in the 1950s and 1960s in parallel with the evolution of the modern pharmaceutical industry.[3] Along with ephedrine and caffeine, anabolic steroids are currently among the most commonly used "performance-enhancing" drugs.[4]

Anti-doping policy and testing of athletes has a relatively short history. Testing, mainly for amphetamines, was gradually introduced during the 1960s. It was not until the 1972 Munich Olympics that a more comprehensive testing programme was carried out at an Olympic Games.[4] This led to seven athletes being disqualified.

In February 1999, the International Olympic Committee hosted a three-day conference in Switzerland to discuss setting up an International Anti-Doping Agency to provide global regulation of drugs in sport. The creation of the agency in time for the 2000 Sydney Olympics was approved as part of a six-point "Lausanne Declaration".

During the 2000 Sydney Olympics, 2846 tests for drugs were carried out, the largest number ever performed during an Olympic

Games. There were 31 positive results. Six of these were pre-prepared "positive" samples to test the quality of the laboratory's work, and 14 were for drugs that had been indicated in a declaration beforehand. Therefore, only 11 of the 31 positive results led to a hearing and a report to the IOC Executive Board.

It is important to note, however, that the use of drugs in sport is not just a problem among elite athletes. There has been growing concern about the use of anabolic steroids by non-competitive sports people.[5]

Regulation

The legal position

At an international level, the Anti-doping Convention of the Council of Europe[6] is the only legally binding document referring to doping, to which there are 32 member country signatories. The convention proposes actions to reduce the trafficking of doping substances, to strengthen doping testing and improve screening programmes, to support education and awareness programmes, and to guarantee the effectiveness of the penalties imposed on offenders.[7]

At the level of the European Union some countries have specific laws on doping, including Austria, Belgium, France, Denmark, Greece, Italy, Portugal, Spain, and Sweden. These laws explicitly forbid doping in sport and contain various measures for prevention and control. Other countries, including the United Kingdom, Germany and The Netherlands, have no specific laws, but rather apply their more general drug laws to the issue. Often this involves legislation, for example on medication, the misuse of drugs, their import, export, and trafficking.[7]

In most countries there are no specific criminal penalties for doping in sport. However, some drugs taken by athletes, such as cocaine and cannabis, are not only banned by the IOC but are also illegal in the UK. Anabolic androgenic steroids (AAS) and anabolic agents such as clenbuterol and polypeptide hormones are designated as class C controlled drugs under the Misuse of Drugs Act 1971. Simple possession is not illegal, unless with intent to supply, and it is an offence to export or import them without an appropriate licence, unless in medicinal form for personal use.

Sporting regulation

At the level of sporting organisations, the Olympic Movement's Anti-Doping Code, Article 1, clearly states that doping contravenes the fundamental principles of Olympism, sports, and medical ethics; that doping is forbidden; and that recommending, proposing, authorising, condoning, or facilitating the use of any substance or method covered by the definition of doping or trafficking therein is also forbidden.

Amateur sports are covered by the same rules as Olympic sports, even though there is a negligible risk of being tested.

In Britain, UK Sport is responsible for carrying out a drug testing and education programme and also works with international agencies to aid the international fight against drugs in sport. Each sport has a regulatory body, called its national governing body (NGB), which is required to maintain an effective anti-doping strategy if it is to receive grants and services from the UK Sports Councils. NGBs must also keep UK Sport informed of their sporting events and indicate which events, teams, and athletes should be prioritised for drug testing.

Each sport also has an International Sports Federation, which is made up of NGBs from each country. To be a member of the International Sports Federation, the NGB must agree to abide by the Federation's regulations. Olympic sports must also comply with the regulations of their country's National Olympic Committee (responsible for their country's Olympic registration). The National Olympic Committee and International Federations of Olympic sports must both abide by the policies of the International Olympic Committee (IOC), the central governing body for Olympic sport.

In 1999 the World Anti-doping Agency was established to coordinate the international anti-doping programme, which is organised at a national level by National Anti-doping Agencies. All International Federations must comply with the regulations of the World Anti-doping Association. The Court of Arbitration for Sport is the main body responsible for arbitration in doping disputes. The IOC set this up, but in recognition of the fact that the Court needed a greater degree of independence from the IOC, the International Council of Arbitration for Sports was created and appoints arbitrators to the Court. Although the IOC cannot appoint arbitrators to the Court it does appoint members of the International Council.

Guidance for doctors

The General Medical Council advises that: "Doctors who prescribe or collude in the provision of drugs or treatment with the intention of improperly enhancing an individual's performance in sport would be contravening the GMC's guidance, and such actions would usually raise a question of a doctor's continued registration. This does not preclude the provision of any care or treatment where the doctor's intention is to protect or improve the patient's health."[8]

The World Medical Association's declaration on Principles of healthcare for sports medicine[9] states: "The Physician should be aware that the use of doping practices by a physician is a violation of the medical oath and the basic principles of the WMA's Declaration of Geneva, which states: 'My patient's health will always be my first consideration'. The WMA considers the problem of doping to be a threat to the health of athletes and young people in general as well as being in conflict with the principles of medical ethics."

The role and responsibilities of doctors are discussed in Chapter 7.

Sporting ethics

There are many ethical issues to address when considering the use of drugs in sport. Some commentators believe that sport should always be drug free; others believe that there is a place for doping as long as it is done under medical supervision and does not damage the health of the competitor. An independent multidisciplinary body, the European Group on Ethics in Science and New Technologies,[7] concluded that there is no place for doping in sport, and outlined a number of issues to consider:

- Doping in sport not only threatens to damage sport as a social institution, it is detrimental to fundamental ethical values which are meant to be at the basis of modern sport, namely fair play and team spirit, or more generally integrity and solidarity.
- The protection of the health of the athlete is also an ethical concern, for it is endangered by the enormous pressure on the athlete to push towards ever higher levels of performance, in the context of sport as a global and commercial enterprise.
- Doping in sport touches on problems of medical ethics, as sports doctors today are called upon to help enhance sports performance by offering medical substances and specific methods for more than simply therapeutic reasons, and in a way which is not readily transparent.
- The doping issue is critical in the case of young and consequently vulnerable sports people, who are involved in intensive training that can damage their health and create psychological dependence.

The main arguments in favour of drug-free sport and an anti-doping policy are therefore as follows: doping is a threat to sport as a social institution; doping is a threat to health and a problem for medical ethics; and doping is a threat to young people.

Doping as a threat to sport as a social institution

This argument considers that drug-taking in sport undermines the values of fair play and the concept of a level playing field. This view, however, is hard to maintain when we consider the inequalities in financial sponsorship and medical expertise available to athletes. Is it possible to believe in a level playing field in the world of professional sport, when we consider that "low-friction swimsuits, the Lotus-designed cycle and the use of aerodynamically designed helmets, skis and ski sticks have all, at various times, conferred a generally acknowledged advantage upon those able to gain initial access"?[4]

Some legitimate practices to improve performance include[10]:

- Endurance training
- Weight training
- Massages
- Anti-inflammatory medications such as aspirin, ibuprofen, and naproxen
- Surgeries for musculoskeletal problems
- Altitude training
- Skills-development training
- Flexibility training.

There is also concern that doping in sport may send out "unhealthy" messages to young people, that it is OK to cheat using potentially harmful drugs. Young athletes may find it particularly difficult to resist drug-taking if it becomes part of the culture of sport as a social institution.

Doping as a threat to health and a problem for medical ethics

One of the arguments for banning drugs in sport is a perception that bans protect the health of the athlete. This may seem uncontroversial. However, if drugs are banned because they are harmful to health, then we also need to consider the health consequences of competing in elite-level athletics. For example, it has been argued that most cyclists who use drugs in the Tour de France do so simply to complete the punishing schedule of the race, not to win. Therefore, should we be arguing that the race should be less strenuous as a strategy to combat drug use? We should not forget that sport itself can carry a risk of death and permanent disability.[4]

The issue of protecting an athlete's health is further confused because natural performance-enhancing techniques are not banned but could equally put the athlete's health at risk. Many athletes use a process of carbohydrate loading, whereby an athlete depletes glycogen stores in an intensive seven-day training session, then consumes a protein-rich diet, then for the remaining three days before competition consumes a starch- and sugar-rich diet to maximise glycogen stores in the muscles. Health consequences of this can include hypoglycaemia, nausea, fatigue, dizziness, and irritability.[11]

The emphasis of anti-doping policies in the UK in recent years has been on punishing those who fail drugs tests. This may appear to protect the health of the athlete. However, it has been argued that the ban increases health risks to athletes by denying users access to medical advice and causing them to turn to high-risk "black market" sources.[12]

Athletes frequently turn to the medical profession to obtain advice on optimum diet, and the use of supplements and drugs. As discussed in Chapter 5, there is an argument that sport has become increasingly "medicalised", and this may also contribute to the problem.[13] Athletes often take a large number of supplements under medical supervision, but this may send out the message that there are pharmacological solutions to training needs, and it may be a short step for an athlete from vitamin pills and supplements to a banned substance.

Doctors who work with drug users at sports clinics advocate a harm reduction policy, and may provide advice on how to use banned drugs safely, which compounds should absolutely not be mixed, and how to reduce risk from bloodborne infections associated with injections.[14] Doctors may consider that "protecting the health of the athlete" requires an educational approach, rather than a necessarily prohibitive one. A policy of prohibition may produce unintentional effects that may work against the stated desire to protect the health of the athlete.

Doping as a threat to young people

It may be argued that professional sports people, by virtue of their chosen profession, are role models, and therefore those who are cheating may send out the wrong signals to young people. However, this same argument is not applied so rigorously to other potential role models for the young, especially from the music industry, television, and cinema. "The fact that many musicians, dancers and television and cinema stars have admitted to using drugs does not lead to a condemnation of their performance in the way that Ben Johnson's Olympic run was condemned."[4]

The viewpoint of the athlete

Often in discussions about drugs in sport, the viewpoint of the athlete is ignored. However, when considering ways to minimise harm and reduce drug abuse, it is necessary to try to understand the athlete's motivation.

The few studies that have been conducted to understand athletes' views on the issue of doping provide a confusing message. On the one hand, the desire to win is powerful and can take second place to health concerns: many athletes report that they would take drugs in certain circumstances. A survey of over 100 top American athletes in the late 1970s revealed that nearly 55% of them reported they would be willing to take a drug which would kill them within a year if it could assure them of an Olympic gold medal.[15] A follow-up to this study in 1984 of 198 world-class athletes found that 52% of them would take a wonder drug that would probably kill them within five years, if it guaranteed success.[16]

On the other hand, athletes appear to be unsympathetic towards fellow athletes who take banned substances. For example, a survey of professional athletes[17] found that although they did not appear to support harsh penalties for first offences which may have been part of an over-the-counter medical treatment for a common ailment, 30% did support a life ban for a second offence. Their attitudes towards those who are caught "positive" for anabolic steroids, amphetamines, or blood doping were much harsher, with 51% supporting a life ban. Of the 48.8% who did not support a life ban for these offences, 49% subsequently stated that they would support a life ban for a second offence of this nature.

A more recent study by the British Olympic Association surveyed British athletes following the 2000 Sydney Olympic Games.[18] When asked to comment on suitable penalties for athletes testing positive for banned substances, many athletes supported strong measures, mentioning life bans and zero tolerance. They found that 26% of athletes felt they did not get adequate information about banned or permitted drugs, or about testing procedures. The earlier study showed that the majority of the athletes questioned (94%) thought that an anti-doping education programme aimed at young competitors would be an effective intervention in reducing future drug use.

However, athletes do not train and compete in isolation. They are part of both an internal group, comprising coach, masseur, physiotherapist, medical practitioners, parents, team mates, and so forth, and an external group comprising their sponsors, their club, sports federations, the media, spectators, and governments. The pressure to meet the expectations of both these groups is great, and conflicts of interest are possible.[7] Verroken[3] has listed the pressures faced by contemporary athletes, which may include:

- Media pressure to win
- Prevalent attitude that doping is necessary to be successful
- Public expectations about national competitiveness
- Huge financial rewards for winning
- Desire to be the best in the world, and to become famous
- Performance-linked payments to athletes from governments and/or sponsors
- Coaching which emphasises winning as the only goal
- Unethical practices condoned by national and international sports federations
- Competitive character of the athlete
- Infallibility of the medical profession to cure and improve performance
- Psychological belief in aids to performance – "the magic pill"
- Development of spectator sport
- Crowded competition calendar.

Unfortunately, anti-doping policies have to date been focused solely on the athletes to the exclusion of these internal and external group members who play a large part in the potential for drug use by the athlete.

References

1 Goldman B, Klatz R. *Death in the Locker Room II*. Chicago: Elite Sports Medicine Publications, 1992.
2 World Health Organization Programme on Substance Abuse. *Drug use and sport: Current issues and implications for public health*. Geneva: WHO, 1993.
3 Verroken M. Drug use and abuse in sport. In: Mottram, DR ed. *Drugs and sport*, 2nd edn. London: E&FN Spon, 1996.

4 Houlihan B. *Dying to win: doping in sport and the development of anti-doping policy.* Strasbourg: Council of Europe, 1999.
5 Korkia P, Stimson GV. *Anabolic steroid use in Great Britain: An exploratory investigation.* The Centre for Research on Drugs and Health Behaviour. A report for the Department of Health, the Welsh Office and the Chief Scientist Office, Scottish Home and Health Department, 1993.
6 Council of Europe. *Anti-doping Convention.* Strasbourg, 1989.
7 European Group on Ethics in Science and New Technologies. *Opinion on the ethical aspects arising from doping in sport.* Brussels, November 1999.
8 British National Formulary Number 41. London: BMA and RPSGB, 2001.
9 World Medical Association. *Principles of health care for sports medicine.* 51st WMA General Assembly, Tel Aviv, Israel, 1999.
10 Salazar A. *Locating the line between acceptable performance enhancement and cheating.* Duke Conference, 1999.
11 Vernacchia RA. Ethical issues of drug use in sport. In: Tricker R, Cook DL eds. *Athletes at risk: Drugs and sport.* Dubuqe IA: Wm C Brown, 1990.
12 Black T. Does the ban on drugs in sport improve societal welfare? *Int Rev Sociol Sport* 1996;**31**:367–80.
13 Waddington I. *Sport, health and drugs.* London and New York: E&FN Spon, 2000.
14 Coomber R. Drugs in sport: Rhetoric or pragmatism. *Int J Drug Policy* 1993;4: 169–78.
15 Donohue T, Johnson N. *Foul play: Drug abuse in sports.* Oxford: Basil Blackwell, 1986.
16 Goldman B, Bush P, Klatz R. *Death in the locker room.* London: Century Publishing, 1984.
17 Radford P. Drug testing and drug education programs. *Science Periodical on Research and Technology in Sport (Coaching Association of Canada)* 1992;**12**: 1–5.
18 British Olympic Association. *Athletes Commission report: Sydney 2000 Olympic Games.* London: BOA, 2001.

3: The medical consequences of taking performance-enhancing and other drugs in sport

Introduction

The International Olympic Committee (IOC) published its first list of banned doping classes in 1967, in which it listed narcotic analgesics, sympathomimetic amines, psychomotor stimulants, and miscellaneous central nervous system stimulants. Since that time the list has evolved and grown, with the incorporation of anabolic steroids in 1974, β blockers and diuretics in 1985, and peptide hormones in 1989. The current (September 2001) IOC list is shown in Table 3.1.

A copy of the IOC list is published in the chapter on "Guidance on Prescribing" in the British National Formulary,[1] which is updated every six months. A more detailed version of the current IOC list, including examples of banned substances and limits on levels of drugs in the urine, where appropriate, can be found on the IOC website: www.olympic.org.

Individual sports federations may devise their own rules concerning doping within their own sport. However, in general these federations follow the guidelines laid down by the IOC Medical Commission.

Drugs may be used by competitors for a number of reasons. These include:

- Therapeutic purposes (prescription drugs or self-medication)
- Performance continuation (treatment for sports injuries)
- Recreational drug use (legal and illegal)
- Performance enhancement.

In each of these categories there are classes of drugs that appear in the IOC list of banned substances. It is important that healthcare professionals are aware of this when prescribing, dispensing over-the-counter

Table 3.1 IOC prohibited classes of substances and prohibited methods 2001–2.

I Prohibited classes of substances
A Stimulants
B Narcotics
C Anabolic agents
1. Anabolic androgenic steroids
2. β-2 agonists
D Diuretics
E Peptide hormones, mimetics and analogues
1. Chorionic gonadotrophin
2. Pituitary and synthetic gonadotrophins (luteinising hormone)
3. Corticotrophins (adrenocorticotrophic hormone, tetracosactide)
4. Growth hormone
5. Insulin-like growth factor (and all the respective factors and their analogues)
6. Erythropoietin
7. Insulin
II Prohibited methods
1. Blood doping
2. Administering artificial oxygen carriers or plasma expanders
3. Pharmacological, chemical and physical manipulation
III Classes of substance prohibited in certain circumstances
A Alcohol
B Cannabinoids
C Local anaesthetics
D Glucocorticosteroids
E β-Blockers

drugs, or offering advice to athletes on medication. Bearing in mind the diverse nature of the circumstances in which athletes may take drugs, advice may include how to take medicines, which medicines to avoid during competition or training, the legal regulations concerning drug use, or the consequences to health if drugs are taken during exercise and in doses in excess of those recommended therapeutically.

The IOC Medical Commission publishes an Anti-Doping Code[2] which intends to ensure respect for sport ethics and to protect the health of the athletes. It is this aspect of the health of the athletes to which this chapter is dedicated. An overview of each of the major classes of drugs and methods banned by the IOC is presented under the headings:

- IOC category
- Potential use in sport

- Pharmacological action
- Adverse effects
- Additional information (where appropriate).

For information, where appropriate drugs are referred to by their Recommended International Non-Proprietary Name, with their British Approved Name appearing in brackets.

The final section of this chapter presents information on therapeutic drugs used in the management of common illnesses that athletes may experience. The adverse effects of these drugs and the implications for their use in sport are described.

IOC prohibited classes of drugs and methods

Amfetamines (amphetamines)

IOC category

I. Prohibited class of substance. A. Stimulants

Potential use in sport

Amfetamines are used during competition to reduce fatigue and to improve reaction time, alertness, competitiveness, and aggression. Amfetamines may be used out of competition to intensify training.

Pharmacological action

There are four mechanisms by which amfetamines may produce their effects.[3] These are:

- By releasing neurotransmitters, such as noradrenaline, dopamine, and serotonin, from their respective nerve terminals
- By inhibition of neurotransmitter uptake
- By direct action on neurotransmitter receptors
- By inhibition of monoamine oxidase activity.

Of these, neurotransmitter release is the most important.

Adverse effects

The adverse effects of amfetamines include restlessness, irritability, tremor, and insomnia, with an increase in aggressive behaviour and the potential for addiction.[4] At higher doses amfetamines may produce sweating, tachycardia, pupillary dilation and increased blood pressure. Effects on the heart may lead to arrhythmias, of which ventricular arrhythmia is potentially fatal.

A particular adverse effect associated with amfetamine misuse in endurance sports such as cycling is heatstroke. Amfetamines produce a redistribution of blood flow away from the skin, thereby impeding the mechanism for reducing body temperature.[5]

Central effects of amfetamines induced by chronic low doses include personality changes which are usually reversed after the drug is withdrawn. However, high chronic usage may lead to an amfetamine psychosis, characterised by psychiatric symptoms commonly found in paranoid-type schizophrenia.[6]

Additional information

Amfetamines and derivatives, such as ecstasy, are recreational drugs, therefore competitors may test positive for amfetamines having not intended to use them for performance enhancement.

Sympathomimetics available in over-the-counter medicines

This group includes drugs such as ephedrine, pseudoephedrine, phenylpropanolamine and phenylephrine.

IOC category

I. Prohibited class of substance. A. Stimulants

The IOC regulations define a positive result for these substances if they appear in the urine at concentrations above 10 or 25 micrograms per millilitre depending on the particular substance.

Potential use in sport

Sympathomimetics cause vasoconstriction, with a concomitant increase in blood pressure. However, they also cause central stimulant effects. It has been suggested[7] that athletes, particularly female bodybuilders, may be disposed to use ephedrine because it promotes fat loss.

Pharmacological action

These drugs are used principally as decongestants in over-the-counter (OTC) preparations, such as cold remedies. They exert their effect through stimulation of α-1 adrenoreceptors in vascular smooth muscle, leading to vasoconstriction and a decrease in mucus secretion. These sympathomimetics are structurally related to amfetamine and therefore produce a similar, though weaker, effect on central neurotransmitters to that described previously.

Adverse effects

Over-the-counter sympathomimetics variably produce side effects such as headache, tachycardia, dizziness, hypertension, irritability, and anxiety. At high doses their amfetamine-like effects could lead to mania or psychosis.[8] Severe effects can also include cerebral haemorrhage and stroke.[9] Following concerns about possible risks from strokes, the Food and Drugs Administration in the US has withdrawn cold remedies containing phenylpropanolamine.

A study of the use of ephedrine in female weightlifters[7] showed that most subjects had experienced at least some adverse effects, with 19% displaying ephedrine dependence.

Additional information

Other drugs which are found commonly in OTC medicines, such as antihistamines (for example triprolidine, astemizole), analgesics (for example paracetamol), imidazole decongestants (for example xylometazoline), cough suppressants (for example pholcodine), and expectorants (for example ipecacuanha), are permitted by the IOC. A more complete list is published in the BNF.[1]

Caffeine

IOC category
I. Prohibited class of substance. A. Stimulants

Potential use in sport

Caffeine may be used primarily for its central stimulant effect to improve alertness, reaction time, and attention span. In addition, caffeine may increase the mobilisation and utilisation of fatty acids, leading to a sparing of muscle glycogen.[10,11]

Pharmacological action

Caffeine inhibits the phosphodiesterase group of enzymes, which activate secondary messengers such as cyclic AMP. They act as one of the links between receptor activation and cellular responses. Caffeine also directly antagonises adenosine receptors.

Adverse effects

Mild side effects associated with caffeine include irritability, insomnia, and gastrointestinal disturbances. More severe effects include peptic ulceration, delirious seizures, coma, and superventricular and ventricular arrhythmias.[9] A condition known as caffeinism has been described by Greden,[12] characterised by symptoms including anxiety, mood changes, sleep disturbances, and psychological changes. Such patients may experience withdrawal symptoms. Excessive doses of caffeine, up to 10g, can be lethal, causing seizures, tachycardia, or ventricular dysrrythmias.[13]

In one study where caffeine was used in combination with ephedrine, during high-intensity exercise some subjects experienced nausea, although the authors did not consider that this effect was due to the caffeine.[14] This finding was in line with a previous study.[15]

Additional information

Because caffeine is so widely consumed in beverages and is available in some OTC medicines (for levels, see [3]), the IOC permits levels up to 12 micrograms per millilitre in urine.

Cocaine

IOC category
I. Prohibited class of substance. A. Stimulants

Potential use in sport

Studies on the ergogenic effects of cocaine are inconclusive.[3] Cocaine is a "recreational" drug and many instances of positive doping results have arisen from residual levels remaining in the body after recreational use, rather than from an attempt by the athlete to enhance performance. Cocaine is notable for distorting the user's perception of reality, therefore the athlete may perceive enhanced performance where, in reality, a decrease in endurance and strength exists because of the drug.[8]

Pharmacological action

The pharmacological effects of cocaine on the brain are complex and include inhibition of the uptake of various central neurotransmitters, particularly dopamine, causing an euphoric effect.

Adverse effects

The complex pharmacology of cocaine leads to a wide spectrum of adverse effects, including a negative effect on glycogenolysis, paranoid psychosis, seizures, hypertension, and myocardial toxicity, which could lead to ischaemia, arrhythmias, and sudden death, especially following intense exercise.[10,16] Smoked "crack" cocaine is more dangerous as the rate of absorption is greater, leading to a more intense effect on the cardiovascular system.[13]

Some bizarre fatalities have been linked to the concomitant use of cocaine with alcohol and anabolic steroids, which may have resulted in the production of a novel cardiotoxic metabolite, norcocaine.[17]

Additional information

Other local anaesthetics are permitted in sport, when medically justified and subject to certain restrictions, principally relating to their route of administration. However, cocaine is excluded from these provisions.

β_2 Agonists

IOC category

I. Prohibited class of substance. A. Stimulants and C.2 Anabolic agents (β_2 agonists)

Potential use in sport

All β_2 agonists are potent bronchodilators and may, therefore, improve performance in aerobic exercise. The significant rise in the number of American Olympic competitors diagnosed with exercise-induced asthma, from 10% in 1984 to 60% in 1994, would suggest that athletes are convinced of the performance-enhancing properties of β_2 agonists.[18] At the 2000 Sydney Olympic Games, 607 (approximately 6%) out of around 10 300 competitors gave notification that they needed to take β_2 agonists. This compares with the UK National

Asthma Audit of 1999/2000 which estimated that around 1 in 25 (4%) of adults (16 years and over) had asthma symptoms requiring treatment. Following the Sydney Olympic Games, the IOC Medical Commission set up a specialist group to investigate the overuse of inhaled β_2 agonists.

Salbutamol, salmeterol, terbutaline, and eformoterol (formoterol) are permitted by inhaler to prevent and/or treat asthma and exercise-induced asthma. Written notification by a respiratory or team physician is required. As from the Winter Olympic Games in Salt Lake City, athletes will be required to submit to the IOC Medical Commission clinical and laboratory evidence (including respiratory function tests) to justify treatment. The evidence must be received at least one week before the athlete first competes. A panel of scientific and medical experts will review the submitted evidence. A letter from the athlete's GP will no longer suffice.

β_2 Agonists, particularly clenbuterol, possess anabolic activity and are used as an alternative or in addition to anabolic steroids. For bodybuilders, clenbuterol is used more for its fat utilising properties, leading to a lean "cut" appearance.

For salbutamol, the definition of a positive test result under the IOC anabolic agent category is determined by a concentration in urine >1000 nanograms per millilitre. As a stimulant, the cut-off level is >100 nanograms per millilitre of urine.

Pharmacological action

Bronchodilation is mediated through stimulation of the β_2 adrenoreceptors in the smooth muscle of the respiratory tract.

β_2 adrenoreceptors are also found in skeletal muscle, stimulation of which induces muscle growth.[19] β_2 agonists are also capable of reducing subcutaneous and total body fat.

Adverse effects

β_2 agonists are selective, not specific, to the β_2 adrenoreceptors. At the higher doses likely to be experienced by misusers in sport, these drugs lose their selectivity, leading to stimulation of β_1 adrenoreceptors. This commonly produces fine tremor, usually of the hands, and may produce tachycardia, arrhythmias, nausea, insomnia, and headache.[20] These side effects are more likely to be experienced following administration by injection or orally.

When clenbuterol is used in doses producing anabolic effects, additional side effects such as generalised myalgia, asthenia, periorbital pain, dizzy spells, nausea, vomiting, and fever have been reported.[21]

Additional information

Other drugs used in the treatment of asthma, including corticosteroids (subject to restriction, see below), anticholinergics, methyl xanthines, and cromoglycate, are permitted in sport.

Narcotics

IOC category
I. Prohibited class of substance. B. Narcotics

Potential use in sport

Potent narcotic analgesics are misused in sport for their pain relieving properties. Certain less potent and permitted narcotics may be used as OTC medications for the management of cough (for example pholcodine, dextromethorphan) and diarrhoea (for example codeine, diphenoxylate).

Pharmacological action

Alkaloids from the opium poppy and their synthetic analogues interact with the receptors in the brain which are normally acted upon by the endogenous endorphin transmitters. They have the capacity to moderate pain but also affect emotions. Frequent use may induce tolerance and dependence, the extent of which is variable depending on the narcotic used.

Adverse effects

In high doses narcotic analgesics can cause stupor and coma, with the possibility of death due to respiratory depression. Where dependence has occurred, withdrawal symptoms include craving, anxiety, sweating, insomnia, nausea and vomiting, muscle aches, and potential cardiovascular collapse.[22]

The use of narcotics to suppress pain may tempt an injured athlete to continue to compete, thereby exacerbating a potentially serious condition.

Additional information

Codeine was removed from the IOC list of banned substances in 1993 as a consequence of the high number of positive test results arising from its availability as an OTC preparation. In 1994 dihydrocodeine and dextromethorphan were similarly deregulated.

Anabolic androgenic steroids

IOC category

I. Prohibited class of substance. C. 1. Anabolic agents (anabolic androgenic steroids)

Potential use in sport

Anabolic androgenic steroids (AAS) are used to improve strength by increasing lean body mass, decreasing body fat, prolonging training by enhancing recovery time, and increasing aggressiveness and energy.

Table 3.2 Some commonly used AAS and testosterone esters.

Dianabol (Methandrostenolone)	Testosterone cypionate
Deca-Durabolin (Nandrolone Decanoate)	Testosterone propionate (Virormone)
Anavar (Oxandrolone)	Testosterone blend (Sustanon 250)
Primobolan (Methenolone)	Testosterone heptylate (Theramex)
Anadrol (Oxymetholone)	Testosterone enanthate (Testaviron)
Anapolon (Oxymetholone)	Testosterone undecanoate (Andriol)
Masteron (Drostanolone)	
Equipose (Boldenone) – a veterinary steroid	
Fluoxymesterone (Halotestin, Ultandren)★	
Norethandrolone (Nilevar)★	
Oxymetholone (Anadrol, Androyd)★	
Metholone (Primobolin)★	
Methyltestosterone (Android)★	
Stanozolol (Winstrol)★	
Methandrostenolone (Dianabol)★	

★ 17α–alkylated androgens.

Polydrug use with AAS is common[23,24] (see Chapter 4). This may be undertaken to enhance anabolic effects (for example with clenbuterol, human growth hormone, human chorionic gonadotrophin), to minimise adverse effects (for example with diuretics, antioestrogens, opiates, corticosteroids, stimulants with anorexic effects), or to increase training intensity (stimulants).

Pharmacological action

AAS have two major effects:
- An anabolic or tissue building effect
- An androgenic or masculinizing action.

Despite efforts to dissociate the two, all anabolic steroids have, to varying degrees, some androgenic effects and are thus recognised as anabolic androgenic steroids. The androgenic effects are often viewed as undesirable owing to their virilising effects, which are especially evident in children and women. They may be taken orally or by deep intramuscular injection. Injectable preparations may be water or oil based. In general, oil-based preparations have a longer biological half-life.

AAS produce their effect through an action on endogenous androgen receptors. They increase protein synthesis and possibly have an anticatabolic effect by antagonising the effect of glucocorticoid hormones such as cortisol, released during intense exercise.[25] Their anticatabolic effects have been demonstrated on patients with severe burn injuries.[26]

Dehydroepiandrosterone (DHEA) is a hormone produced by the adrenal glands and serves as a precursor in the endogenous production of androgens and oestrogens, including androstenedione, testosterone and dihydrotestosterone. It may also increase the levels of insulin-like growth factor-1 (IGF-1).[27] DHEA is therefore banned by the IOC.

Adverse effects

There are a number of adverse effects associated with AAS, many potentially serious. For reviews, see WHO[22] and Tucker.[28]

The incidence of adverse effects due to AAS could be expected to be high, as they are frequently used in doses 10–30 times higher than needed for replacement therapy, and multiple steroid regimens, such as stacking and pyramiding, are commonly used.[29] Up to five steroids were identified in urine samples from bodybuilders in one study.[30] That AAS are commonly used in cycles of on-AAS and off-AAS is likely to dampen the degree of adverse effect. AAS-related adverse effects are often considered under six main headings: cardiovascular, cosmetic, hepatic, infections, reproductive, and psychiatric. Although systematic life-threatening side effects have not been substantiated in the available medical literature, there is a total lack of prospective studies of the long-term effects of AAS exposure on mortality. In other words, much of the evidence of AAS effects is based on case studies and speculation about risk factor effects, such as raised high-density lipoprotein (HDL) levels. Common methodological problems with studies concerning AAS use include small sample sizes, lack of controls, failure to confirm exposure and to consider the veracity of self-reports, and failure to account for confounding factors, such as other drug use, weight training, and free testosterone levels (Buchan, I, personal communication 2001). The effects and interactions of the range of preparations commonly taken by users, including "recreational" and "black market" drugs, make it difficult to assess possible health outcomes.

Cosmetic effects: Acne, particularly on the back, and water retention are common reversible side effects in both sexes. Prolonged use may lead to male-pattern baldness. Gynaecomastia is a common side effect among male bodybuilders and is associated with steroid use.[31,32] Physicians have been approached by athletes with a view to obtaining tamoxifen to prevent this condition[33] and surgery to treat it.[32] The risks of steroid use in women are greater than in men, with irreversible cosmetic effects in particular.[34,35] Females tend to prefer oral steroids, which are shorter acting than the oil-based injected preparations such as testosterone. Testosterone is more likely to produce side effects such as acne, unwanted facial hair, clitoromegaly, and a change in the shape of the face, with squaring of the jaw line.[34] The oral 17α-alkylated androgens are known to be more liver toxic.[36,37] In a study on self-reported side effects for women[38] the most common reports concerned psychological effects, deepening of the voice, and menstrual problems. Other side effects suffered by female AAS users include breast atrophy.

Cardiovascular risk: The cardiovascular risks of AAS use have been highlighted in many studies[39–42] and there is some clinical evidence to suggest that these risks may be considerable. Studies[43] have shown that total cholesterol levels remain unchanged following AAS use, but HDL is reduced in some individuals while low density lipoprotein (LDL) is increased. This may increase the risk of developing atherosclerosis. The HDL lowering effect appears to be confined to 17α-alkylated androgens, as a 50% reduction in HDL levels has been shown.[28,44] Derangement of plasma lipids is rapidly reversed with cessation of use.[45–49]

At present, only speculative evidence resting on risk factor effects and case studies is available on the link between AAS and coronary heart disease. Similarly, evidence for increased platelet aggregation leading to increased coagulation and thrombosis is based on one pilot observational study.[50]

Other associated side effects include cardiomyopathy and stroke. Both are based on speculation from case reports, and the risk of stroke in particular is based on risk factor effects.[39] Thibilin et al.[51] had 34 deceased male AAS users autopsied for medicolegal reasons. They found that in 12 cases chronic cardiac changes were evident. Observational studies of athletes using AAS compared to controls have only lent speculative evidence for the link between cardiomyopathies and AAS use.[52-54] Evidence for systematic hypertension directly attributable to steroids is debatable,[55] and controlled studies in athletes and non-athletes have not detected any significant effects of AAS on blood pressure.[44,56-58] One study has shown significantly impaired glucose tolerance and greater insulin resistance in 15 long-term AAS-using power lifters compared with 6 obese and 10 non-obese sedentary controls,[59] and two other controlled studies showed no significant effects after the administration of testosterone esters.[60,61] Long-term controlled studies are needed to describe the true risks of AAS on the cardiovascular system.

Liver tumours and dysfunction: The liver is a target tissue for androgens and is the principal site for steroid metabolism, especially after oral administration. A number of adverse effects on the liver have been described, including hepatocyte hypertrophy and, at high doses, cholestasis and peliosis hepatis.[37] The two latter conditions have been seen mainly in patients with severe anaemia in response to treatment with 17α-alkylated androgens. AAS use can also result in altered liver enzyme function, especially if 17α-alkylated androgens are used.[62] In a recent case-control study Dickerman et al.[63] found no derangement in liver enzymes in 15 self-administering AAS users compared to non-users, whereas elevations were seen in patients with hepatitis. Androgens may also increase the risk of liver tumours,[64] and they appear to promote tumour function.[65] Generally, men are at a greater risk of developing liver cancer than are women. In the literature, there are 21 case reports of liver tumour regression when 17α-alkylated androgens were withdrawn in patients prescribed AAS for severe anaemia or hypogonadism, or misuse of AAS. Distinctive pathological features of liver tumours in patients taking AAS have led pathologists to describe a distinct androgen-sensitive neoplasm of the liver.[36] Anabolic androgenic steroid users should therefore be cautioned about the serious medical consequences of taking these drugs.

Reproductive effects: In males, AAS use is associated with testicular atrophy, reduced sperm production, and changes in sperm motility. Testosterone esters induce reversible azoospermia in normal men, and their efficacy as a male contraceptive has been accepted by the WHO.[57] Interviews with AAS users have revealed that they commonly take human growth hormone (hCG) towards the end of a cycle to stimulate endogenous testosterone production following exogenous androgen use, partly to avoid testicular atrophy.[31,66] Similarly, in women AAS users amenorrhoea has been reported by up to 80%.[38,67] There are no reports in the literature of irreversible reproductive effects on men or women who have used AAS, even for extended periods. More seriously, prostatic cancer has been induced in the animal model with AAS,[68] although in humans controlled studies have not linked AAS use with the condition.[57,61,69]

Infections: In addition to the pharmacological side effects of AAS, complications may result from the injection techniques used by self-administrators.[70] Injecting AAS use has been linked with HIV, AIDS, hepatitis, and myobacterial infection in bodybuilders.[71–73] British data suggest that there may be a danger of spreading bloodborne infections; Perry[74] noted that 31 out of 45 new clients in a needle exchange service (NXS) in Wales admitted having shared injecting equipment. The danger of sharing may be substantial, as a quarter of 110 interviewees said that their friends mainly injected them.[66] Anecdotal reports of macho "shotgunning" techniques, that is, injecting both buttocks simultaneously, are of concern. The potential problems of sharing vials and dividing drugs using syringes have been highlighted by Midgley *et al.,*[75] who interviewed 50 AAS users and 40 non-users in London. They found that needle sharing was not common practice, but 19% had shared multidose vials and 17% had divided AAS doses using syringes, both being potential routes for HIV and hepatitis infection if injectors reused injecting equipment.

"Irresponsible" sexual behaviour is also a potential route for the transmission of infections: Midgley *et al.*[75] found that an increase in sex drive was more commonly reported by AAS users, and more AAS users also engaged in sex with more than one partner but used condoms infrequently. However, there is no direct evidence in the literature of a higher seroprevalence of HIV, hepatitis B or C in AAS users.

How strong is the evidence for life-threatening effects of AAS?

The incidence of death or life-threatening diseases associated with AAS use has so far been relatively low, and has largely been linked with long-term and high-dose use. Although it may well be that the occurrence of life-threatening events really is rare, it is also possible that effects are not reported because AAS use may not be considered as a possible cause by practitioners, and patients do not always volunteer the information.[76] It is also possible that their effects may only emerge later in life, as suggested by the Parssinen *et al.* study.[77]

Apart from the female-to-male transsexual conversion studies where high-dose androgen therapy is applied,[78,79] there is an acute lack of long-term prospective studies of high-dosage AAS use as it is taking place. Attempts to convince AAS users of serious adverse effects in the absence of convincing data have had the effect of alienating them from the medical profession.[80,81] A number of case studies have linked AAS use to sudden death,[82–84] but although valuable information can be derived from such studies, the resulting perceived associations between AAS and any particular condition cannot have the same status as associations derived from controlled studies. In a 12-year follow up study by Parssinen *et al.*[77] a cohort of 62 previously highly competitive power lifters who were *suspected* of AAS use were compared to controls. They reported a high incidence of premature deaths and mortality: 12.9% of the power lifters compared to 3.1% in the control population. This study highlights the potential health dangers of AAS use. Thibilin *et al.*[51] provided a slightly stronger case for the implications of AAS use when they found that of the 34 autopsies performed on AAS users, 12 had chronic cardiac changes. However, in the current situation, where polydrug use is the norm, a direct cause-and-effect relationship may be very difficult to prove.

A public health physician has recently compiled a critical review to assess the evidence of AAS-related harm (Buchan I, personal communication 2001). Among the 364 related abstracts, more than half were rejected because they were case reports, anecdotes, or uncontrolled studies. It was found that *strong* evidence of causation for AAS and specific pathologies only existed for reduced HDL to LDL count, reversible male infertility, virilisation of females, and truncal acne. *Acceptable* evidence exists for androgen-sensitive liver neoplasia, gynaecomastia, dependence, and increase in risk behaviours for sexually transmitted diseases. In this category, evidence for AAS-related aggression was found to be non-significant or very small and significant. Buchan highlighted the lack of prospective long-term studies of AAS use, and especially the lack of information about cardiovascular risks. As this review shows, the literature on AAS is limited, to a large extent, to non-controlled, observational, case and cross-sectional studies. Hence, it is difficult at the moment to draw firm conclusions about AAS-related harm, and lack of evidence should not be interpreted as evidence for an absence of harmful adverse effects.

Psychological effects

Psychological effects with AAS, such as mania, hypomania, and depression, have been reported.[85] The effects have consistently been shown not to be uniform across users, even with relatively high dose administration.[58,86,87] An interesting study with a relatively high dose of testosterone enanthate (600mg weekly) injections did not find any differences in emotional state, mood, anger, and partner perceptions before, during, or after AAS administration.[88] Tricker *et al.*[89] showed no significant effects on anger and mood in a double-blind randomised placebo-controlled trial, and Yates *et al.*,[90] in a similarly controlled trial, found no effects on aggression and psychosexual behaviour.

In contrast, Su *et al.*[58] found a dose–effect relationship for both positive and negative mood, mood swings, violent feelings, anger and hostility, and cognitive symptoms, with a 240mg daily dose of methyltestosterone. They reported, however, that the effects were highly variable in their small ($n = 20$) sample of non-athletic men. Further, they found no link between plasma androgen levels and symptoms recorded. Williamson[91] has speculated on the effects of expectations on the psychiatric outcomes with AAS use. He points out that some actually hope that AAS will make them aggressive, and this is what many users also state. On the other hand, Williamson[91] speculates that those who are already aggressive by nature may be more inclined to use them: indeed, abnormal personality traits have been shown more often in AAS users than in controls.[92]

Aggression, health, and safety: The actual influence of AAS on behaviour is an important issue from the public health and safety perspective; however, it is also an immensely complicated one. The sensitivity to certain AAS, interactions of heavy training, extreme dieting, polypharmacy, including psychostimulant use, "black market" preparations, prior personality dimensions, and expectations are likely to potentiate their effects, but also make an assessment of the AAS effects on mood and behaviour extremely complicated. In Britain, the new "arrest–referral" schemes apparently do not include AAS in the list of drugs offenders are asked about, and valuable information about the issue of AAS use and criminality is therefore lost.

AAS use has been associated with mood changes, antisocial, aggressive, and violent behaviour, and its possible role as a precursor to violent crime has been highlighted.[31,58,66,93–98] Currently, it is not known whether a cause-and-effect relationship exists between AAS use and domestic violence and/or violent crime.[87] In the early 1990s, the Metropolitan police reported five cases of AAS-linked violent crimes, including rape and murder (Bristow C, personal communication 1992). Choi and Pope[97] reported in a cross-sectional intrasubject study of 23 AAS-using and 14 non-using athletes that periods of AAS use were characterised by significantly greater levels of verbal aggression and violence than periods of non-use. AAS use has been reported to result in accidental death, suicide in predisposed individuals, and becoming a victim of a homicide.[51,99] Thirteen per cent of AAS users in one study reported "always, very often or often" having urges to "beat, injure and harm" others while taking AAS, whereas only 4% felt this way when off AAS.[66] Lenehan et al.[31] reported that 31% of their sample of 386 AAS users experienced urges to harm others while on AAS. It is not known to what extent these urges were translated into action, for example in domestic situations.

Dependence: Dependence on AAS has been reported.[100–104] For example, Tennant et al.[102] induced opioid-like withdrawal symptoms in an AAS user who felt addicted to them. The symptoms included fatigue and depression. The study by Brower et al.[101] of 49 AAS-using US male weightlifters revealed that 57% met the criteria for dependence. Dependent users took higher doses and more cycles, and reported significantly more dissatisfaction with body size than non-dependent users. Four other cross-sectional studies using the same criteria for dependence have reported rates between 14% and 69% in AAS-using US weightlifters.[85,104–106]

Tennant et al.[102] and Kashkin and Kleber[103] suggested that AAS may affect the endogenous opioid or monoaminergic systems in the brain, to produce dependence, discontinuation depression, and suicidal ideation. However, it may simply be the feeling of wellbeing and the better physique resulting from the use of AAS that provides the psychological stimulus to continue their use.[28] In 1991, Brower et al.[101] showed that dissatisfaction with body image may represent a psychological vulnerability that predisposes AAS takers to dependence. The fact that the majority of AAS users are capable of periods off AAS (cycling) supports the evidence that they may be addictive only to selected users, or to those taking high doses. In AAS users the proposed mechanism of dependence involves two systems:

- Positive reinforcement: brain reward system similar to opioid use and/or improved self-esteem and social standing owing to impressive musculature
- Negative reinforcement: avoidance of depression and/or withdrawal symptoms, and loss of muscle mass.

The clinical evidence of dependence on AAS in some users is supported by evidence of a withdrawal syndrome in the animal model.[107]

Other effects: Evidence for the effects of AAS-induced tendon damage is inconclusive and the speculation arises from animal studies and case reports.[108,109] AAS use accompanied by exercise may lead to dysphasia of collagen fibrils, which can decrease the tensile strength of tendons. Changes in tendons' crimp morphology have been shown to occur, which may alter the rupturing strain of tendons.[110] However, strenuous exercise itself produces excessive loading on the tendon.

For ethical reasons, no scientific experiments have been conducted on the effects of AAS in adolescents. However, it has been predicted that adolescents risk the same adverse effects as seen in adults, with the additional possibility of growth arrest,[111] which is probably irreversible.[35] Concern also centres on the establishment of normal endocrine function. Data from studies of growth arrest have generally reported minor side effects.[112,113] Because these studies are characterised by low doses, a direct comparison with self-administration of AAS is not feasible. The possibility of young people being more vulnerable in terms of cardiovascular and carcinogenic outcomes has been raised.[114]

Additional information

Anabolic androgenic steroids (AAS) and anabolic agents such as clenbuterol and polypeptide hormones are designated as class C controlled drugs under the Misuse of Drugs Act 1971.

Diuretics

IOC category

I. Prohibited class of substance. D. Diuretics

Potential use in sport

Diuretics do not have performance-enhancing effects, but have been used to increase urine production in an attempt to dilute other doping agents and/or their metabolites. This form of manipulation is unlikely to be effective.[115] Diuretics are also used to reduce weight in sports where weight classification applies. In this context, athletes are subject to testing at the time of the weigh-in. Diuretics may also be used by female athletes, for example in gymnastics, dancing, and figure skating, for weight loss or to manage premenstrual fluid retention.[116]

Pharmacological action

Diuretics variably exert their pharmacological effect on the kidney, to produce an increased loss of fluid. All pharmacological classes of diuretics are banned by the IOC.

Adverse effects

In virtually all studies where diuretic usage during exercise has been evaluated, deleterious effects have been reported.[117] The primary effect results from induced hypohydration, although concomitant electrolyte disturbances, such as changes in potassium levels, compromise the heart and muscles. These effects are exacerbated where hyperthermia and dehydration accompany fatigue and glycogen depletion.

Where diuretics are used to attain a lower weight classification, the length of time between the weigh-in and the competition is crucial in determining the potential adverse effects on performance and health.

Additional information

Diuretics are used by bodybuilders to counteract the fluid retentive effects of androgenic anabolic steroids.

Human growth hormone

IOC category

I. Prohibited class of substance. E. 4. Growth hormone

Potential use in sport

Similarly to AAS, human growth hormone (hGH) is used to increase muscle mass, to allow users to train harder, longer, and more frequently, and to promote faster recovery after training.

Pharmacological action

Human GH is a polypeptide hormone produced by the pituitary gland to maintain normal growth from birth to adulthood. It has a short (about 20 minutes) half-life, during which time it activates hepatic GH receptors, mediating the production of insulin-like growth factor-1 (IGF-1). It is IGF-1 that is responsible for most of the anabolic action of hGH.[118]

Adverse effects

Overuse of hGH in children can lead to "gigantism", in adults it can lead to "acromegaly".[119] Features of acromegaly include skeletal deformities, arthritis, and enlargement of organs such as the heart, lungs, liver, intestines, and spleen. Hypertension, diabetes mellitus, peripheral neuropathy, and muscle weakness, despite an increase in size, may develop. Increased protein synthesis also produces thickening and coarsening of the skin. Mortality is high, with 50% of patients with acromegaly dying before the age of 50, and 89% dying before the age of 60, of heart failure.[120] The changes associated with acromegaly are not likely to occur in the majority of athletes using hGH as they use the drug for short periods of time, with long breaks between use, and in doses lower than those seen in acromegalic patients.[121] Associations between the use of hGH and certain cancers have been reported. The only positive correlation seems to be with leukaemia.[122]

Evidence for the adverse effects of hGH in sport is sparse. Short-term abuse with hGH produces acute fluid retention.[123] In two studies on the effects of hGH in athletes,[124,125] 2 out of 18 and 3 out of 11 subjects, respectively, withdrew from the study with carpal tunnel compression. In the second of these studies, four of the subjects experienced oedema of the fingers, which resolved despite continued treatment with hGH.

A study of the mechanical properties of the skin of bodybuilders who were abusing recombinant hGH showed that although skin deformability and biological elasticity remained within the normal range, an increase in dermal viscosity was noted.[126]

Before 1986, hGH was freeze-extracted from the pituitaries of human cadavers. This has led to the risk that recipients may contract Creutzfeldt–Jakob disease (CJD), secondary to viral contaminants. As there is an average 15-year incubation interval, exposed athletes may not yet have undergone the requisite incubation period.[127] Currently, recombinant hGH is the preparation of choice, although cheaper, cadaveric hGH is still available on the "black market".

Where athletes use IGF-1, adverse effects are the same as for hGH. IGF-1 commonly produces hypoglycaemia, as it promotes the uptake of glucose into cells.[27]

Additional information

The use of hGH has become more popular among female athletes, as there is no risk of developing the androgenic side effects associated with AAS.[128]

Erythropoietin

IOC category

I. Prohibited class of substance. E. 6. Erythropoietin

Potential use in sport

The increase in production of erythrocytes by erythropoietin (EPO) improves the oxygen carrying capacity of the blood. This effect is particularly useful in endurance sports. Misuse normally involves synthetic recombinant EPO (rEPO).

Pharmacological action

EPO is a glycoprotein hormone produced primarily in the kidney. The stimulus for its production is reduced oxygen delivery to the kidney. Its effect is to increase the number of erythrocytes that are produced from the bone marrow and to increase the rate at which they are released into the circulation.[129] It has been shown that the time to exhaustion and increase in $VO_{2\,max}$ (maximum oxygen intake) using EPO is similar to that obtained with blood reinfusion.[130]

Adverse effects

EPO can, initially, produce flu-like symptoms, such as headaches and joint pain, but these usually resolve spontaneously, even with continued use. Up to 35% of patients on EPO develop hypertension, and the risk of thrombosis is increased.[131]

In sport, the misuse of EPO poses a significant potential risk to health, as the raised haematocrit increases blood viscosity, which may be further exacerbated through dehydration. At haematocrit levels above 55% there is a substantial risk of coronary or cerebral artery occlusion. It has been suggested that the unusually high number of deaths of competitive cyclists in The Netherlands and Belgium between 1987 and 1990 was associated with EPO use.[132]

There is little published research on the use of EPO by athletes. One study[133] on the short-term effects of rEPO, using 20 subjects, revealed no adverse effects over a 24-day period. At the end of the 24-day period, blood pressure levels were no different from initial values and no convulsive or thrombolytic events were recorded. However, Ekblom[134] has reported that whereas blood pressure after EPO was unaltered at rest, there was a marked increase in the systolic blood pressure of subjects during submaximal exercise.

Additional information

The IOC introduced a testing procedure for EPO for the first time at the Sydney Olympic Games in 2000. The procedure comprised two tests, an electrophoretic test on urine samples to distinguish recombinant EPO from endogenous EPO, and a blood test to characterise erythrocytes, because rEPO produces macrocytic and hypochromic red cells. EPO levels can also be increased by training at high altitudes or using a hypobaric oxygen chamber.[116] A modified test is currently being developed.[135]

Other peptide hormones

This category includes human chorionic gonadotrophin (hCG), luteinising hormone (LH), adrenocorticotrophic hormone (ACTH), and insulin.

IOC category
I. Prohibited class of substance. E. Peptide hormones, mimetics and analogues

Insulin is permitted only to treat athletes with certified insulin-dependent diabetes. Written certification must be obtained from an endocrinologist or team physician. As with other peptide hormones, proving that an athlete has used insulin illicitly is very difficult.

Potential use in sport

These peptide hormones are used to potentiate the endogenous levels of other hormones with ergogenic or other performance-enhancing properties.

Pharmacological action

Endogenous levels of testosterone may be increased by the use of hCG and LH. ACTH increases adrenal corticosteroid release. hCG stimulates testicular steroidogenesis, especially testosterone, without upsetting the testosterone/epitestosterone ratio,[136] therefore the IOC test criteria for testosterone would not be triggered. A recent review[137] has suggested that, in addition to facilitating glucose entry into cells, insulin increases muscle bulk through inhibition of muscle protein breakdown.

Adverse effects

There is little published research on the effects of these hormones in athletes. Side effects of hCG include oedema (particularly in males), headache, tiredness, mood changes, and gynaecomastia. Adverse effects of ACTH are related to released glucocorticoids. Although insulin is being used increasingly by competitors, to date there have been no published reports on its adverse effects in athletes.

Prohibited methods

This category comprises:

1. Blood doping
2. Administering artificial oxygen carriers or plasma expanders
3. Pharmaceutical, chemical, and physical manipulation.

IOC category

II. Prohibited methods

Potential use in sport

Blood doping increases the oxygen carrying capacity of the blood. Manipulation includes the use of drugs (for example probenecid, epitestosterone) to mask the use of other doping agents, or the use of physical means (for example urine substitution) to avoid detection.

Pharmacological action

Probenecid may delay the excretion of other doping agents, such as anabolic androgenic steroids. Epitestosterone is used to maintain the ratio of testosterone to epitestosterone in the urine within IOC accepted limits (less than or equal to 6:1).

Adverse effects

Blood doping may lead to adverse effects associated with hyperviscosity of the blood, as discussed under EPO. Otherwise, autologous blood doping carries no more risk than any other procedure involving invasive techniques. However, risks due to cross-infection and non-matched blood may occur where homologous infusion is carried out, especially without medical supervision.[134]

Alcohol

IOC category
III. Classes of prohibited substances in certain circumstances. A. Alcohol

Potential use in sport

Alcohol (ethyl alcohol) may potentially be used as a performance-enhancing drug because of its anti-anxiety effect. In some team sports, where alcohol is part of a social convention, peer pressure may lead to overindulgence, with consequences for the partaker and for fellow competitors.

Pharmacological action

Alcohol affects neural transmission in the central nervous system (CNS) by altering the permeability of axonal membranes and thereby slowing nerve conduction. Alcohol also decreases glucose utilisation in the brain. Overall, alcohol impairs concentration, reduces anxiety, and induces depression and sedation.[138]

Adverse effects

The adverse effects of alcohol have been extensively documented over many centuries.

Cannabinoids

IOC category
III. Classes of prohibited substances in certain circumstances. B. Cannabinoids

Potential use in sport
Cannabinoid effects are incompatible with most sports, therefore tests are only conducted in certain sports. Despite this, the number of positive results for marijuana from IOC testing laboratories continues to rise, and the consequences for the user and their fellow competitors need to be reviewed.[139]

Pharmacological action
The active constituent of marijuana is 1-5-9-tetrahydrocannabinol (THC). When smoked, 60–65% is absorbed and effects are noted within 15 minutes and last for 3 hours or more.[138] It produces a sedating and euphoric feeling of wellbeing.

Adverse effects
The central depressant effects of THC decrease the motivation for physical effort and motor coordination, and short-term memory and perception are also impaired. In addition to its psychological effects, THC induces tachycardia, bronchodilation, and an increased blood flow to the limbs.[138]

Additional information
Passive smoking of cannabinoids has been cited as the reason for a positive test result on a number of occasions, most notably at the Winter Olympic Games at Nagano, in February 1998. As a consequence, the IOC has recently introduced a clause that states that a urine concentration of the metabolite carboxy-THC of less than 15 nanograms per millilitre does not constitute doping at Olympic Games.

Local anaesthetics

IOC category
III. Classes of prohibited substances in certain circumstances. C. Local anaesthetics

Local anaesthetics are permitted in sport provided they are medically justified and written notification is presented. The route of administration is restricted to local or intra-articular injection.

Potential use in sport

Local anaesthetics may be used to treat minor sporting injuries.

Pharmacological action

Local anaesthetics act by causing a reversible block to conduction along nerve fibres.

Adverse effects

Little information has been published on the adverse effects of local anaesthetics in sport.

Additional information

Cocaine is banned for use as a local anaesthetic in sport.

Glucocorticosteroids

IOC category

III. Class of prohibited substance in certain circumstances. D. Glucocorticosteroids

Topical administration of glucocorticosteroids is permitted if the route of administration is limited to perianal, aural, or skin application. Inhalation, nasal or ophthalmological routes, or local or intra-articular injection, are also permitted. Written notification of administration may be required by some sport federations. The systemic use of glucocorticosteroids is prohibited when administered orally, rectally, or by intravenous or intramuscular injection.

Potential use in sport

Glucocorticosteroids are important in the management of sports injuries because of their potent anti-inflammatory properties.

Pharmacological action

These drugs are related to the adrenocorticosteroid hormone released from the adrenal cortex. They have a widespread effect on the body, including glucocorticoid effects on carbohydrate, protein and fat metabolism, and on electrolyte and water balance, as well as their anti-inflammatory effect. As anti-inflammatory agents they reduce the swelling, tenderness, and heat associated with injury by reducing the output of the biochemical mediators of inflammation and by inhibiting the responsiveness of white blood cells.[140]

Adverse effects

As with analgesics, the chronic or prolonged use of corticosteroids to reduce pain and swelling, thereby allowing the athlete to continue to compete, may lead to an exacerbation of an injury, possibly leading to osteoporosis.

Local damage may be produced at the site of injection owing to dosage volume and subcutaneous atrophy, with associated depigmentation, telangiectasia and striae. Although atrophy and depigmentation may be reversible after several years, fat atrophy and striae are usually permanent.[141] Corticosteroids produce a catabolic effect on skeletal muscle, leading to muscle weakness soon after treatment has begun, even with modest doses.

Fredberg,[142] in a review of local corticoid injection in sport, states that injection of corticosteroid inside the tendon has a deleterious effect on the tendon tissue and should be avoided, but that there is no reliable proof of the deleterious effect of corticosteroid with peritendinous injection. Fredburg[142] also provides guidelines for local injection therapy with corticosteroids.

Systemic complications with corticosteroids include transient hyperglycaemia in people with diabetes, vasovagal attack, psychological problems, and systemic allergic reactions.[143]

A significant adverse effect with long-term systemic corticosteroid treatment is the suppressant effect on the output of endogenous glucocorticosteroid from the adrenal cortex. Sudden withdrawal of corticosteroid treatment may leave the adrenal gland unable to respond to the demand for glucocorticosteroid. Gradual withdrawal of treatment is therefore required.

β blockers

IOC category

III. Class of prohibited substance in certain circumstances. E. β blockers

Potential use in sport

β blockers have a potential use in sport where motor skills can be affected by muscle tremor caused by anxiety. β blockers are therefore prohibited in certain sports, such as archery and other shooting events, and in high-risk sports such as ski jumping, bobsleigh, and luge. A full list of Olympic events in which β blockers are banned is published by the IOC (www.olympic.org).

Pharmacological action

β adrenoreceptors are widely distributed throughout the body, and so consequently the pharmacology of β blockers is complex. They are first-line drugs in the management of angina pectoris, hypertension, some cardiac arrhythmias, hyperthyroidism, and glaucoma, and are used occasionally for migraine and essential tremor. Three subclasses of β adrenoreceptors are recognised as being clinically significant. The selectivity of β blockers for these subclasses is important in determining their therapeutic action and potential side effects.

Adverse effects

The adverse effects of β blockers vary according to the properties of the individual drug. These drugs may induce bronchospasms or cause insomnia, nightmares, and depression.[116] β blockers which are cardio-selective are less likely to induce bronchoconstriction. Those with intrinsic sympathomimetic activity are less likely to produce fatigue and cold extremities, and those which are more lipophilic can more readily cross the blood–brain barrier and are more likely to produce sleep disturbances and nightmares. It is unlikely that β blockers would be used in sport in doses greater than those used therapeutically.

Additional information

β blockers were reclassified by the IOC in March 1993, from class I to class III, reflecting their limited use in certain sports.

Therapeutic drugs in the management of illness

In this section, consideration is given to the use of therapeutic drugs in the management of illnesses that athletes may experience and for which they may self-medicate or seek medical advice from a general practitioner, pharmacist, or other healthcare professional.

A useful review of this subject is presented by Henderson,[144] who raises the following questions for the athlete's prescriber:

1. Does the diagnosis really require medication? Is non-pharmacological management appropriate? Is the condition self-limiting?
2. Can the potential adverse effects of the medication be minimised through consideration of the most appropriate dose and route of administration?
3. Is the chosen medication banned by the athlete's sport's governing body?
4. Should the athlete compete while ill?

With these questions in mind, some of the more commonly used drugs are presented below.

Non-steroidal anti-inflammatory drugs

Potential use in sport

Non-steroidal anti-inflammatory drugs (NSAIDs) are widely used as analgesic and anti-inflammatory drugs for the treatment of sports injuries. One famous ex-England cricketer has been quoted as saying that "players have been accustomed to using these drugs as though they were sweets".[145] They are not banned by the IOC. Leadbetter[146] suggests that when first encountering the injured athlete the physician should ask four basic questions: 1) Is the problem serious? 2) Will continued sports participation cause harm? 3) How can the patient be rid of the problem? 4) When can play resume? If pain and signs of inflammation are persistent, repeated attempts to turn off the body's alarm system can place an athlete in jeopardy with respect to tissue overload and failure.

Pharmacological action

The analgesic, anti-inflammatory, and antipyretic activity of NSAIDs is based on their ability to inhibit prostaglandin synthesis. In addition, aspirin and other NSAIDs inhibit the synthesis of thromboxane, thereby inhibiting platelet aggregation. This property has been put to therapeutic advantage in the prevention of the development of thromboses.

Adverse effects

The most common adverse effects associated with NSAIDs are gastrointestinal, including nausea, dyspepsia (in up to a third of patients), and ulcers (1–2% of patients). However, caution needs to be exercised regarding polydrug use in sport.

NSAIDs exhibit other side effects and should be avoided in athletes with a known allergy to these drugs, with a history of bleeding disorders, and with compromised renal or liver functions.[147] Hypersensitivity reactions to NSAIDs are more likely to occur in asthmatics and in individuals prone to chronic rhinitis or chronic urticaria.

Although corticosteroid injection therapy is often regarded by the patient as the more extreme measure, an oral NSAID can carry a far greater systemic risk.[146] There are suggestions that the use of NSAIDs may not hasten the return of injured athletes back to competition.[148]

Additional information

Topical administration of NSAIDs may offer an effective and possibly safer alternative route of administration.[149,150] An even safer alternative is available through topical rubefacients.

Muscle relaxants

Potential use in sport

There are a number of drugs, such as benzodiazepines and dantrolene sodium, which have muscle relaxant effects. They are not generally recommended for the treatment of athletic injury. Further information on benzodiazepines is given below.

Anxiolytics

Potential use in sport

Competing in sport instils various psychological reactions, including anxiety. A moderate level of anxiety about a forthcoming event is deemed desirable to induce the right levels of motivation for action, but high levels of anxiety militate against performance.[138] A number of classes of drugs have been used as anxiolytics, including alcohol, β blockers, and benzodiazepines. The first two classes have already been described above, as they are restricted in certain sports.

Pharmacological action

Benzodiazepines variously reduce the activity of a number of central neurotransmitters, such as acetylcholine, serotonin and noradrenaline. The anti-anxiety effect is primarily through the release of γ-aminobutyric acid, which inhibits the release of serotonin.

Adverse effects

Benzodiazepines are relatively free of adverse effects. However, they are liable to produce dependence if used for extended periods, which is unlikely in the case of athletes. Benzodiazepines may also be used by athletes for insomnia. Under these circumstances, athletes need to be aware of the "hangover" effect of these drugs. The shorter-acting compounds, such as lorazepam and oxazepam, are preferable under these circumstances.

Cough and cold preparations

Potential use in sport

The use of medication for these self-limiting conditions is questionable. The underlying cause is viral in nature and does not warrant antibiotic treatment. The only potential use for drugs is for the control of symptoms such as headache, fever, runny nose, and cough. However, many of the drugs found in OTC cough and cold remedies, particularly the α-1 sympathomimetic decongestants, are banned by the IOC, although there are cut-off concentrations in the urine for these drugs (see above). Nonetheless, competitors run the risk of testing positive and being banned for using these drugs.

Pharmacological action

Apart from the sympathomimetic decongestants discussed previously, cough and cold medicines may contain analgesics (paracetamol, codeine), antihistamines (for example triprolidine, astemizole), imidazole decongestants (for example xylometazoline), cough suppressants (for example pholcodine), and expectorants (for example ipecacuanha), all of which are permitted by the IOC.[151]

Adverse effects

In general, cough and cold preparations are taken for short periods of time and therefore side effects are limited. However, nasal decongestants are liable to produce rebound congestion if used for more than one week. Sedating antihistamines may have adverse effects on performance in most sports.

Antidiarrhoeals

Potential use in sport

Athletes, like non-athletes, are liable to experience acute diarrhoea. First-line treatment is oral rehydration therapy (ORT). Antimotility drugs may be used for short-term symptomatic relief of acute diarrhoea if it is likely to affect performance.

Pharmacological action

ORT enhances the absorption of water and replaces electrolytes. It contains alkalinising agents to counter acidosis. Antimotility drugs (codeine, diphenoxylate, loperamide, morphine) are opioids with a direct relaxant effect on the smooth muscle of the gastrointestinal tract.

Adverse effects

Tolerance and dependence may develop with prolonged use of antimotility drugs. Loperamide may produce abdominal cramps, drowsiness, and skin reactions.

Additional information

Apart from morphine, the opioid antimotility drugs are permitted by the IOC.

Nutritional supplements

Potential use in sport

In an attempt to enhance performance through ergogenic aids without contravening IOC regulations, many athletes have used nutritional supplements.[139]

There is limited legal control on the content of nutritional supplements, and in 2000 there were a number of high-profile cases regarding positive test results involving nandrolone, where the athletes claimed that the nandrolone found in their urine must have been present in nutritional supplements that they had used.

Pharmacological action

Unlike therapeutic drugs, nutritional supplements are not required to have strong scientific and clinical evidence that they are effective before being allowed to be sold to the public.[152] Manufacturers may therefore make exaggerated claims regarding the ergogenic properties of their products.[153] There is little, if any, evidence that nutritional supplements possess ergogenic properties in athletes consuming a balanced diet.

Adverse effects

Some nutritional supplements have the potential for harm.[153] Studies in which diet was manipulated to induce metabolic acidosis, by reducing carbohydrate intake or increasing fat and protein intake, have shown impaired performance.[154]

Concern has been expressed that young adults may be consuming vast quantities of nutritional supplements. Creatine has been the subject of many studies, but results are equivocal as to whether it produces ergogenic effects.[152,155,156] There are few reliable scientific data on the possible adverse effects of creatine. Kayne[157] has reported that the potential effect on renal dysfunction and electrolyte imbalance, leading to a predisposition to dehydration and heat-related illness, suggests caution in its use. On the other hand, Schilling et al.[158] have concluded that their studies show that their subjects' kidney function tests all fell within the normal range.

Anecdotal reports of creatine supplementation causing gastrointestinal problems have been refuted by Kreider et al.[159] who, in a retrospective analysis of five of their published studies, found that reports of gastrointestinal distress were isolated and fewer than for subjects on placebo. Long-term use of high doses of creatine is not recommended[160] especially in athletes with recognised renal dysfunction.[161]

Other therapeutic agents, such as tamoxifen and thyroxine, are used as supplements by anabolic steroid abusers, as discussed in the next chapter.

Additional information

UK Sport warns that supplements represent an unknown risk for athletes, as the products are not subject to stringent regulatory and licensing requirements or controlled by a specific organisation. Hence, it is difficult to determine whether all the constituents have been listed on the packaging, or whether the composition would vary without notice. For this reason, UK Sport and governing bodies cannot give a "definitive response to requests about the status of these products". Athletes should think seriously about whether they are really necessary to achieve a genuine performance, with supplements being taken at the athlete's own risk. Ideally, they should not be taken at all.[161]

Summary

This chapter has aimed to set out information about which drugs and doping methods are used by sports people for what reasons, and what adverse effects may be encountered as a result of this. In addition, information about other drugs, not banned by the IOC but which athletes may require, has been outlined, explaining any effects that they might have on the athlete's performance. It is hoped this may assist prescribers and their patients through the potentially confusing regulations, and highlight the potentially serious medical consequences and powerful adverse effects of drug use for non-medical purposes in sport.

References

1 *British National Formulary.* London: BMA and RPSGB, 2001.
2 International Olympic Committee Medical Commission. *Olympic movement anti-doping code.* IOC, 1999.
3 George A. Central nervous system stimulants. In: Mottram DR, ed. *Drugs in sport, 2nd edn.* London: E&FN Spon, 1996 .
4 Knopp WD, Wang TW, Bach BR. Ergogenic drugs in sports. *Clin Sports Med* 1997;**16**: 375–92.
5 Rosenbloom D, Sutton JR. Drugs and exercise. *Med Clin North Am* 1985;**69**: 177–87.
6 Connell PH. *Amphetamine psychosis.* London: Chapman & Hall, 1958.
7 Gruber AJ, Pope HG. Ephedrine abuse among 36 female weightlifters. *Am J Addiction* 1998;7: 256–61.
8 Schwenk TL. Psychoactive drugs and athletic performance. *Phys Sports Med* 1997;**25**: 32–46.
9 Wadler GA, Hainline B. *Drugs and the athlete.* Philadelphia: Davies Company, 1989.
10 Conlee RK. Amphetamine, caffeine and cocaine. In: Gisolfi CV, Lamb DR, eds. *Perspectives in exercise science and sports medicine.* New York: Brown and Benchmark, 1991.

11 Dodd SL, Herb RA, Powers SK. Caffeine and exercise performance: An update. *Sports Med* 1993;**15**: 14–23.
12 Greden JF. Anxiety or caffeinism: a diagnostic dilemma. *Am J Psychiatry* 1974;**131**: 1089–92.
13 Ghaphery NA. Performance-enhancing drugs. *Orthop Clin North Am* 1995;**26**: 433–42.
14 Bell DG, Jacobs I, Zamecnik J. Effects of caffeine, ephedrine and their combination on time to exhaustion during high-intensity exercise. *Eur J Appl Physiol Occup Physiol* 1998; 77:427–33.
15 Graham TE, Spriet LL. Metabolic, catecholamine and exercise performance responses to various doses of caffeine. *J Appl Physiol* 1995;**78**: 867–74.
16 Eichner ER. Ergolytic drugs in medicine and sports. *Am J Med* 1993;**94**: 205–11.
17 Welder AA, Melchert RB. Cardiotoxic effects of cocaine and anabolic-androgenic steroids in the athlete. *J Pharmacol Toxicol Meth* 1993;**29**: 61–8.
18 Eichner ER. Ergogenic aids: what athletes are using and why. *Phys Sports Med* 1997;**25**: 70–9.
19 Yang YT, McElligott MA. Multiple actions of βadrenergic agonists on skeletal muscle and adipose tissue. *Biochem J* 1989;**261**: 1–10.
20 Prather ID, Brown DE, North P, Wilson JR. Clenbuterol: a substitute for anabolic steroids? *Med Sci Sports Exercise* 1995;**27**: 1118–21.
21 Meyer HHHD. Anabolic β-agonists: biochemistry of action, pharmacokinetics, adverse effects in man and control in urine and blood. *Blood samples in doping control.* Oslo: Pensumtjeneste (On Demand Publishing), 1994.
22 World Health Organization. *Drug use and sport. Current issues and implications for public health.* Geneva: WHO, 1993.
23 Korkia P. Anabolic-androgenic steroids and their uses in sport and recreation. *J Substance Misuse* 1997;**2**: 131–5.
24 Evans NA. Gym and tonic: a profile of 100 male steroid users. *Br J Sports Med* 1997;**31**: 54–8.
25 Marone JR, Falduto MT, Essig DA, Hickson RC. Effects of glucocorticoids and endurance training on cytochrome oxidase expression in skeletal muscle. *J Appl Physiol* 1994;77: 1685–90.
26 Sheffield-Moore M. Androgens and the control of skeletal muscle protein synthesis. *Ann Med* 2000;**32**: 181–6.
27 Sturmi JE, Diorio DJ. Anabolic agents. *Clin Sports Med* 1998;**17**: 261–82.
28 Tucker R. Abuse of anabolic-androgenic steroids by athletes and bodybuilders: A review. *Pharm J* 1997;**259**: 171–9.
29 Mottram DR, George AJ. Anabolic steroids. *Best Practice Res Clin Endocrinol Metab* 2000;**14**: 55–69.
30 Delbeke FT, Desmet N, Debackere M. The abuse of doping agents in competing bodybuilders in Flanders (1988–1993). *Int J Sports Med* 1995;**16**: 66–70.
31 Lenehan P, Bellis M, McVeigh J. Anabolic steroid use in the North West of England. *J Performance Enhancing Drugs* 1996;**1**: 57–70.
32 Reyes RJ, Zicchi S, Hamed H, Chaudary MA, Fentiman IS. Surgical correction of gynaecomastia in bodybuilders. *Bri J Clin Prac* 1995;**49**: 177–9.

33 Salaman JR. Misuse of anabolic drugs. *BMJ* 1993;**306**: 6869.
34 Honour JW. Steroid abuse in female athletes. *Curr Opin Obstet Gynaecol* 1997;**9**: 181–6.
35 Wu FCW. Endocrine aspects of anabolic steroids. *Clin Chem* 1997;**43**: 1289–92.
36 Anthony PP. Liver tumours. *Baillières Clin Gastroenterol* 1988;**2**: 501–22.
37 Friedl KE. Effects of anabolic steroids on health. In: Yesalis CE, ed. *Anabolic Steroids in Sport and Exercise*. Campaigne: Human Kinetics Publishers Inc., 1993.
38 Korkia P, Lenehan P, McVeigh S. Non-medical use of androgens among women. *J Performance Enhancing Drugs* 1996;**1**: 71–6.
39 Mochizuki RM, Richter KJ. Cardiomyopathy and cerebrovascular accident associated with anabolic-androgenic steroid use. *Phys Sports Med* 1988;**16**: 109–14.
40 Stolt A, Karila T, Viitasalo M, Mantysaari M, Kujala U, Karjalainen J. QT interval and QT dispersion in endurance athletes and in power athletes using large doses of anabolic steroids. *Am J Cardiol* 1999;**84**: 364–6.
41 Kuipers H, Wijnen J, Hartgens F, Willems S. Influence of anabolic steroids on body composition, blood pressure, lipid profile and liver functions in bodybuilders. *Int J Sports Med* 1991;**12**: 413–18.
42 McCarthy K, Tang AT, Dalrymple-Hay MJ, Haw MP. Ventricular thrombosis and systemic embolism in bodybuilders: Etiology and management. *Ann Thorac Surg* 2000;**70**: 658–60.
43 Glazer G. Athrogenic effects of anabolic steroids on serum lipid levels. *Arch Intern Med* 1991;**151**: 1925–33 .
44 Friedl KE, Hannan CJ Jr, Jones RE, Plymate SR. High-density lipoprotein cholesterol is not decreased if an aromatizable androgen is administered. *Metabolism* 1990;**39**: 69–74.
45 Costill D, Pearson D, Fink W. Anabolic steroid use among athletes: Changes in HDL-C levels. *Phys Sports Med* 1984;**12**: 113–7.
46 Hurley BF, Seals DR, Hagberg JM *et al.* High-density-lipoprotein cholesterol in bodybuilders v powerlifters. Negative effects of androgen use. *JAMA* 1984;**252**: 507–13.
47 Peterson GE, Fahey TD. HDL-C in five athletes using anabolic-androgenic steroids. *Phys Sports Med* 1984;**12**: 120–30.
48 Webb OL, Laskarzewski PM, Glueck CJ. Severe depression of high-density lipoprotein cholesterol levels in weight lifters and bodybuilders by self-administered exogenous testosterone and anabolic-androgenic steroids. *Metabolism* 1984;**33**: 971–5.
49 Lenders JW, Demacker PN, Vos JA *et al.* Deleterious effects of anabolic steroids on serum lipoproteins, blood pressure, and liver function in amateur bodybuilders. *Int J Sports Med* 1988;**9**: 19–23.
50 Ferenchick GS, Kirlin P, Potts R. Steroids and cardiomyopathy. How strong a connection? *Phys Sports Med* 1991;**19**: 107–10.
51 Thibilin I, Lindquist O, Rajs J. Cause and manner of death among users of anabolic androgenic steroids. *J Forensic Sci* 2000;**45**: 16–23.
52 Salke RC, Rowland TW, Burke EJ. Left ventricular size and function in bodybuilders using anabolic steroids. *Med Sci Sports Exercise* 1985;**17**: 701–4.

53 Yeater R, Reed C, Ullrich I, Morise A, Borsch M. Resistance trained athletes using or not using anabolic steroids compared to runners: effects on cardiorespiratory variables, body composition, and plasma lipids. *Br J Sports Med* 1996;**30**: 11–14.

54 Zuliani U, Bernardini B, Catapano A, Campana M, Cerioli G, Spattini M. Effects of anabolic steroids, testosterone, and hGH on blood lipids and echocardiographic parameters in bodybuilders. *Int J Sports Med* 1989;**10**: 62–6.

55 Riebe D, Fernhall B, Thompson PD. The blood pressure response to exercise in anabolic steroid users. *Med Sci Sports Exercise* 1992;**24**: 633–7.

56 Cable NT, Todd L. Coronary heart disease risk factors in bodybuilders using anabolic steroids. *J Performance Enhancing Drugs* 1996;**1**: 25–8.

57 World Health Organization Task Force on Methods for the Regulation of Male Fertility. Contraceptive efficacy of testosterone-induced azoospermia in normal men. *Lancet* 1990;**336**: 955–9.

58 Su ST, Pagliano M, Schmidt PJ, Pickar D, Wolkowitz O, Rubinow DR. Neuropsychiatric effects of anabolic steroids in male normal volunteers. *JAMA* 1993;**269**: 2760–5.

59 Cohen JC, Hickman R. Insulin resistance and diminished glucose tolerance in powerlifters ingesting anabolic steroids. *J Clin Endocrinol Metab* 1987;**64**: 960–3.

60 Matsumoto AM. Effects of chronic testosterone administration in normal men: safety and efficacy of high dosage testosterone and parallel dose-dependent suppression of luteinizing hormone, follicle-stimulating hormone, and sperm production. *J Clin Endocrinol Metab* 1990;**70**: 282–7.

61 Swerdloff RS, Palacios A, McClure RD, Campfield LA, Brosman SA. Male contraception: Clinical assessment of chronic administration of testosterone enanthate. *Int J Androl* 1978;**2**(Suppl): 731–47.

62 Alen M, Rahkila P, Marniemi J. Serum lipids in power athletes self-administering testosterone and anabolic steroids. *Int J Sports Med* 1985;**6**: 139–44.

63 Dickerman RD, Pertusi PM, Zachariah NY, Dufour DR, McConathy WJ. Anabolic steroid-induced hepatotoxicity: Is it overstated? *Clin J Sports Med* 1999;**9**: 34–9.

64 Creagh TM, Rubin A, Evans DJ. Hepatic tumours induced by anabolic steroids in an athlete. *J Clin Pathol* 1988;**41**: 441–3.

65 Lesna M, Taylor W. Liver lesions in BALB/C mice induced by an anabolic androgen (Decadurabolin), with and without pretreatment with diethylnitrosamine. *J Steroid Biochem* 1986;**24**: 449–53.

66 Korkia PK, Stimson GV. *Anabolic Steroid Use in Great Britain: an exploratory investigation.* The Centre for Research on Drugs and Health Behaviour. A report for the Department of Health, the Welsh Office and the Chief Scientist Office. Scottish Home and Health Department, 1993.

67 Strauss RH, Liggett MT, Lanese RR. Anabolic steroid use and perceived effects in ten weight-trained women athletes. *JAMA* 1985;**253**: 2871–3.

68 Noble RL. Androgen use by athletes: a possible cancer risk. *Can Med Assoc J* 1984;**130**: 549–50.

69 Cooper CS, Perry PJ, Sparks AE, MacIndoe JH, Yates WR, Williams RD. Effect of exogenous testosterone on prostate volume, serum and semen

prostate specific antigen levels in healthy young men. *J Urol* 1998;**159**: 441–3.

70 Evans NA. Local complications of self-administered anabolic steroid injections. *Br J Sports Med* 1997;**31**: 349–50.

71 Scott M, Scott M. HIV infection associated with injections of anabolic steroids. *AMA* 1989;**262**: 207–8.

72 Sklarek H, Mantovani R, Erens E, Heisler D, Niederman M, Fein A. AIDS in a bodybuilder using anabolic steroids. *N Engl J Med* 1984;**311**: 1701.

73 McBride AJ, Williamson K, Petersen T. Three cases of nalbuphine hydrochloride dependence associated with anabolic steroid use. *Br J Sports Med* 1996;**30**: 69–70.

74 Perry H. Counterfeit: Fake anabolic steroids and hazards of their use. *Relay* 1995;**1**: 9–11.

75 Midgley SJ, Heather N, Best D, Henderson D, McCarthy S, Davies JB. Risk behaviours for HIV and hepatitis infection among anabolic-androgenic steroid users. *AIDS Care* 2000;**12**: 163–70.

76 Lloyd FH, Powell P, Murdoch AP. Anabolic steroid abuse by bodybuilders and male subfertility. *BMJ* 1996;**313**: 100–1.

77 Parssinen M, Kujala U, Vartiainen E, Sarna S, Seppala T. Increased premature mortality of competitive powerlifters suspected to have used anabolic agents. *Int J Sports Med* 2000;**21**: 225–7.

78 Lowdell CP, Murray-Lyon IM. Reversal of liver damage due to long term methyltestosterone and safety of non-17α-alkylated androgens. *BMJ* 1985;**291**: 637.

79 Westaby D, Paradinas FJ, Ogle SJ, Randell JB, Murray-Lyon IM. Liver damage from long-term methyltestosterone. *Lancet* 1977;**2**: 262–3.

80 Yesalis CE, Streit AL, Vicary JR, Friedl KE, Brannon D, Buckley W. Anabolic steroid use: Indications of habituation among adolescents. *J Drug Educ* 1989;**19**: 103–16.

81 Morrison CM. Harm reduction with AS users: Experiences in running a well users service. *Relay* 1994;**2**: 16–18.

82 Hausmann R, Hammer S, Betz P. Performance enhancing drugs (doping agents) and sudden death: A case report and review of literature. *Int J Legal Med* 1998;**111**: 261–4.

83 Capasso A. Peliosis hepatis in a young adult bodybuilder. *Med Sci Sports Exercise* 1994;**26**: 2–4.

84 Luke JL, Farb A, Virmani R, Sample RHB. Sudden cardiac death during exercise in a weight lifter using anabolic androgenic steroids: Pathological and toxicological findings. *J Forensic Sci* 1990;**35**: 1441–7.

85 Pope HC, Katz DL. Psychiatric and medical effects of anabolic-androgenic steroid use. *Arch Gen Psychiatry* 1994;**51**: 375–82.

86 Brower KJ. Assessment and treatment of anabolic steroid withdrawal. In: Yesalis CE, ed. *Anabolic Steroids in Sport and Exercise*. Campaigne: Human Kinetics Publishers Inc., 1993.

87 Pope HG Jr, Kouri EM, Hudson JI. Effects of supraphysiologic doses of testosterone on mood and aggression in normal men: a randomised controlled trial. *Arch Gen Psychiatry* 2000;**57**: 133–40.

88 Bhasin S, Storer TW, Berman N *et al*. The effects of supraphysiologic doses of testosterone on muscle size and strength in normal men. *N Engl J Med* 1996;**335**: 1–7.

89 Tricker R, Casaburi R, Storer TW *et al.* The effects of supraphysiological doses of testosterone on angry behavior in healthy eugonadal men – a clinical research center study. *J Clin Endocrinol Metab* 1996;**81**: 3754–8.

90 Yates WR, Perry PJ, MacIndoe J, Holman T, Ellingrod V. Psychosexual effects of three doses of testosterone cycling in normal men. *Biol Psychiatry* 1999;**45**: 254–60.

91 Williamson DJ. What are the psychological effects of anabolic steroid use? *Relay* 1994;**1**: 2–3.

92 Cooper CJ, Noakes TD, Dunne T, Lambert MI, Rochford K. A high prevalence of personality traits in chronic users of anabolic-androgenic steroids. *Br J Sports Med* 1996;**30**: 246–50.

93 Pope HG, Katz DL. Homicide and near-homicide by anabolic steroid users. *J Clin Psychiatry* 1990;**51**: 28–31.

94 Copeland J, Peters R, Dillion P. Anabolic-androgenic steroid use disorders among a sample of Australian competitive and recreational users. *Drug Alcohol Dependence* 2000;**60**: 91–6.

95 Pope HG Jr, Kouri EM, Powell KF, Campbell C, Katz DL. Anabolic-androgenic steroid use among 133 prisoners. *Am J Psychiatry* 1996;**153**: 1369.

96 Galligani N, Renck A, Hansen S. Personality profile of men using anabolic androgenic steroids. *Horm Behav* 1996;**30**: 170–5.

97 Choi PYL, Pope HG. Violence toward women and illicit anabolic-androgenic steroid use. *Ann Clin Psychiatry* 1994;**6**: 21–5.

98 Schulte H, Hall M, Boyer M. Domestic violence associated with anabolic steroid abuse. *Am J Psychiatry* 1993;**150**: 348.

99 Thibilin I, Runeson B, Rajs J. Anabolic steroids and suicide. *Ann Clin Psychiatry* 1999;**11**: 223–31.

100 Brower KJ, Blow FC, Elipoulos GA, Beresford TP. Anabolic androgenic steroids and suicide. *Am J Psychiatry* 1989;**146**: 1075.

101 Brower KJ, Blow FC, Young JP, Hill EM. Symptoms and correlates of anabolic-androgenic streroid dependence. *Br J Addiction* 1991;**86**: 759–68.

102 Tennant F, Black DL, Voy RO. Anabolic steroid dependence with opioid-type features. *N Engl J Med* 1988;**319**: 578.

103 Kashkin KB, Kleber HD. Hooked on hormones? An anabolic steroids addiction hypothesis. *JAMA* 1989;**262**: 3166–70.

104 Malone DA, Dimenoff RJ, Lombardo JA, Sample RHB. Psychiatric effects of and psychoactive substance use in anabolic-androgenic steroid users. *Clin J Sports Med* 1995;**5**: 25–31.

105 Gridley D, Hanrahan S. Anabolic-androgenic steroid use among male gymnasium participants: Dependence, knowledge and motives. *Sport Health* 1994;**12**: 11–14.

106 Clancy GP, Yates WR. Anabolic steroid use among substance abusers in treatment. *J Clin Psychiatry* 1992;**53**: 97–100.

107 Bonson K, Garrick N, Murphy D. Evidence for a withdrawal syndrome following chronic administration of an anabolic steroid to rats. *Soc Neurosci Abs* 1994;**20**: 1527.

108 Miles J, Grana W, Egle D, Min K, Chitwood J. The effect of anabolic steroids on the biomechanical and histological properties of rat tendon. *J Bone Joint Surg [Am]* 1992;**74**: 411–22.

109 Michna H. Tendon injuries induced by exercise and anabolic steroids in experimental mice. *Int Orthop* 1987;**11**: 157–62.

110 Laseter JT, Russell JA. Anabolic steroid-induced tendon pathology: A review of the literature. *Med Sci Sports Exercise* 1991;**23**: 1–3.

111 Korkia P. Anabolic steroid use in adolescents. *Sports, Exercise Injury* 1996;**2**: 136–40.

112 Jackson S, Rallison M, Buntin W, Johnson S, Flynn R. Use of Oxandrolone for growth stimulation in children. *Am J Dis Child* 1973;**126**: 481–4.

113 Richman R, Kirch L. Testosterone treatment in adolescent boys with constitutional delay in growth and development. *N Engl J Med* 1988;**319**: 1563–7.

114 Salva PS, Bacon GE. Anabolic steroids and growth hormone in the Texas Panhandle. *Texas Med* 1989;**85**: 43–4.

115 Delbeke FT, Debackere M. The influence of diuretics on the excretion and metabolism of doping agents. *Drug Res* 1986;**36**: 134–7.

116 CASA National Commission on Sports and Substance Abuse. *Winning at any cost: Doping in Olympic sports.* New York: University of Columbia, CASA, 2000.

117 Caldwell JE. Diuretic therapy and exercise performance. *Sports Med* 1987;**4**: 290–304.

118 Russell-Jones DL, Umpleby AM, Hennessy TR *et al.* Use of aleucine clamp to demonstrate that IGF-1 actively stimulates protein synthesis in normal humans. *Am J Physiol* 1994;**267**: E591–8.

119 Healy ML, Russell-Jones D. Growth hormone and sport: Abuse, potential benefits, and difficulties in detection. *Br J Sports Med* 1997;**31**: 267–8.

120 Haupt HA. Anabolic steroids and growth hormone. *Am J Sports Med* 1993;**21**: 468–74.

121 Anon. Use and side effects of growth hormone. *Drugs in Sport* 1992;**1**: 5–7.

122 Fradkin JE, Mills JL, Schonberger LB *et al.* Risk of leukemia after treatment with pituitary growth hormone. *JAMA* 1993;**270**: 2829–32.

123 Wallace JD, Cuneo RC, Lundberg PA *et al.* Response of markers of bone and collagen turnover to exercise, growth hormone (GH) administration and GH withdrawal in trained adult males. *J Clin Endocrinol Metab* 2000;**85**: 124–33.

124 Yarasheski KE, Campbell JA, Smith K, Rennie MJ, Holloszy JO, Bier DM. Effect of growth hormone and resistance exercise on muscle growth in young men. *Am J Physiol* 1992;**262**: E261–7.

125 Deyssig R, Frisch H, Blum WF, Waldhor T. Effect of growth hormone treatment on hormonal parameters, body composition and strength in athletes. *Acta Endocrinol* 1993;**128**: 313–8.

126 Pierard-Franchimon C, Henry F, Crielaard JM, Pierard GE. Mechanical properties of skin in recombinant human growth factor abusers among bodybuilders. *Dermatology* 1996;**192**: 389–92.

127 Anon. Unfavourable clinical events linked directly to contaminants and to the biological actions of growth hormone. *Drugs in Sport* 1994;**2**: 24–7.

128 Ehrnborg C, Bengtsson B, Rosen T. Growth hormone abuse. *Best Practice Res Clin Endocrinol Metab* 2000;**14**: 71–7.

129 Armstrong DJ, Reilly T. Blood boosting and sport. In: Mottram DR ed. *Drugs and sport, 2nd edn.* London: E&FN Spon, 1996.

130 Ekblom BT, Berglund B. Effect of erythropoietin administration on maximal aerobic power. *Scand J Med Sci Sports* 1991;**1**: 88–93.

131 Drug and Therapeutics Bulletin. Epoetin: An important advance. *Drug Ther Bull* 1992;**30**: 29–32.

132 Pena N. Lethal injection. *Bicycling* 1991;**32**: 80–1.

133 Souillard A, Audran M, Bressolle F, Gareau R, Duvallet A, Chanal JL. Pharmacokinetics and pharmacodynamics of recombinant erythropoietin in athletes. Blood sampling and doping control. *Br J Clin Pharmacol* 1996;**42**: 355–64.

134 Ekblom BT. Blood boosting and sport. *Best Practice Res Clin Endocrinol Metab* 2000;**14**: 89–98.

135 UK Sport. Leading journal slams supplements. *UK Sport Press Release 050601*, 2001.

136 Delbeke FT, Van Eenoo P, De Backer P. Detection of human chorionic gonadotrophin misuse in sports. *Int J Sports Med* 1998;**19**: 287–90.

137 Sonksen PH. Hormones and Sport. Insulin, Growth Hormone and Sport. *J Endocrinol* 2001; **170**: 13–25.

138 Reilly T. Alcohol, anti-anxiety drugs and sport. In: Mottram DR, ed. *Drugs in sport, 2nd edn.* London: E&FN Spon, 1996.

139 Mottram DR. Banned drugs in sport. Does the International Olympic Committee (IOC) list need updating? *Sports Med* 1999;**27**: 1–10.

140 Elliott P. Drug treatment of inflammation in sports injuries. In: Mottram DR, ed. *Drugs in sport, 2nd edn.* London: E&FN Spon, 1996.

141 Bentley S. Treatment of sports injuries by local injection. *Br J Sports Med* 1981;**15**: 71–4.

142 Fredberg U. Local corticosteroid injection in sport: review of literature and guidelines for treatment. *Scand J Med Sci Sports* 1997;**7**: 131–9.

143 Leadbetter WB. *Sports-induced inflammation.* Park Ridge Illinois: Am Academy of Orthopaedic Surgeons, 1990.

144 Henderson JM. Therapeutic drugs: What to avoid with athletes. *Clin Sports Med* 1998;**17**: 229–43.

145 Waddington I. *Sport, health and drugs: A critical sociological perspective.* London and New York: E&FN Spon, 2000.

146 Leadbetter WB. Anti-inflammatory therapy in sports injury. The role of non-steroidal drugs and corticosteroid injection. *Clin Sports Med* 1995: **14**: 353–410.

147 Houglum JE. Pharmacological considerations with the treatment of injured athletes with nonsteroidal anti-inflammatory drugs. *J Athletic Training* 1998;**33**: 259–63.

148 Hertel J. The role of non-steroidal anti-inflammatory drugs in the treatment of acute soft tissue injury. *J Athletic Training* 1997;**32**: 350–8.

149 Radermacher J, Jentsch D, Scholl MA, Lustinetz T, Frolich JC. Diclofenac concentrations in synovial fluid and plasma after cutaneous application in inflammatory and degenerative joint disease. *Br J Clin Pharmacol* 1991;**31**: 537–41.

150 Weiler JM. Medical modifiers of sports injury. The use of nonsteroidal anti-inflammatory drugs (NSAIDs) in sports soft-tissue injury. *Clin Sports Med* 1992;**11**: 625–44.

151 Armstrong DJ. Sympathomimetic amines and their antagonists. In: Mottram DR ed. *Drugs in sport, 2nd edn*. London: E&FN Spon, 1996.
152 Clarkson PM. Nutrition for improved sport performance: Current issues on ergogenic aids. *Sports Med* 1996;**21**: 393–401.
153 Beltz SD, Doering PL. Efficacy of nutritional supplements used by athletes. *Clin Pharm* 1993;**12**: 900–8.
154 MacClaren DPM. Alkalinizers: influence of blood acid-base status on performance. *Esteve Foundation Symposium. Vol. 7. The clinical pharmacology of sport and exercise*. Amsterdam: Excerpta Medica, 1997.
155 Balsom PD. Creatine supplementation in humans. *Esteve Foundation Symposium. Vol. 7. The clinical pharmacology of sport and exercise*. Amsterdam: Excerpta Medica, 1997;167–77.
156 Demant TW, Rhodes EC. Effects of creatine supplementation on exercise performance. *Sports Med* 1999;**28**: 49–60.
157 Kayne S. Creatine: the athlete's wonder supplement? *Pharm J* 1999;**263**: 906–8.
158 Schilling BK, Stone MH, Utter A *et al*. Creatine supplementation and health variables: a retrospective study. *Med Sci Sports Exercise* 2001;**33**: 183–8.
159 Kreider RB, Ferreira M, Wilson M *et al*. Effects of creatine supplementation on body composition, strength, and sprint performance. *Med Sci Sports Exercise* 1998;**30**: 73–82.
160 Koshy KM, Griswold E, Schneeberger EE. Interstitial nephritis in a patient taking creatine. *N Engl J Med* 1999;**340**: 814–5.
161 Pritchard NR, Kalra PA. Renal dysfunction accompanying oral creatine supplements. *Lancet* 1998;**351**: 1252–3.
162 UK Sport. Drugs and sport: Herbal and nutritional supplements. In: UK Sports Council *Competitors' and officials' guide to drugs and sport*. London: UK Sport, 1998.

4: Anabolic androgenic steroid use in British gymnasiums

Introduction

Those participating in sports at a recreational non-competitive level, such as gymnasium users, may use techniques and substances, in particular anabolic androgenic steroids (AAS), to enhance their performance or to improve their physique. Research indicates that a third of GPs are likely to encounter patients who have used AAS,[1] and this chapter aims to provide an overview of the problem.

Reports of increasing AAS use among non-competitive groups have been emerging in Australia, Canada, the USA, the UK and the rest of Europe. In 1992 the Departments of Health for England, Scotland and Wales commissioned an investigation into the extent and use of AAS from a public health perspective, resulting in the Korkia and Stimson report.[2] Many of the data in this chapter are based on this extensive British study, and also the comprehensive Northwest study by Lenehan et al.[3]

What are anabolic androgenic steroids?

Anabolic androgenic steroids are a group of synthetic compounds that are structurally related to the natural male hormone testosterone. Male hormones have been used for health purposes since as early as 140 BC, when impotence was treated with the ingestion of animal testes. However, it was not until 1939 that it was suggested that sex hormones might prove useful in improving performance in sport.[4] Five years later, data published from animal and human studies provided support for these speculations. The male hormone testosterone was isolated, and many synthetic compounds, which became known as anabolic steroids, were developed to mimic its effects. A list of commonly used AAS can be found on page 23.

Mechanisms of AAS action

The proposed mechanisms of action of anabolic steroids, allowing a greater volume of training, more frequently and at a greater intensity, without injury or overtraining, is associated with antagonism of the catabolic effects of glucocorticoids (mainly cortisol). This prevents the catabolic state that follows training and instead allows the body to remain in an anabolic state.[5] There is good evidence to show that testosterone and AAS have the potential for increased protein synthesis and muscle mass development.[6] Studies by Demling and Orgill[7] have highlighted their uses in post-traumatic care of burn victims, owing to their ability to stimulate protein synthesis and their anti-catabolic effects.

The central nervous system effects of AAS are proposed to increase motivation and decrease fatigue, thereby maximising effort during the training event.[8,9] As with most drugs, they also have powerful placebo effects. Anecdotal evidence and interview data consistently show that the beneficial effects of AAS are perceived to be substantial in terms of increased muscle mass and size, decreased fat mass, improved performance, intensified training, increased libido, and improved self-confidence.[2,3]

Early scientific studies investigating their efficacy in bringing the desired effects were contradictory, and the reader is referred to reviews and articles for further details.[10-12] Although some well-designed recent studies have shown no improvement with low-dose androstenedione administration,[13] it is worth noting that no study to date has shown a decrement in muscle mass, size, or performance. Reasons for the lack of agreement, especially between older studies, are linked to factors such as small sample sizes, lack of dietary control, variable training status of subjects, differences in the type and dose of drug(s) used, length of use, and the placebo effect.[12] From an ethical perspective, it has been difficult to study high-dose multiple drug use regimens, which are typical for AAS users, in a more controlled fashion.

Demographics of AAS use in gymnasiums

Users of AAS are commonly divided into three main groups:

- "Recreational" bodybuilders, that is, those who train with weights to improve their size and appearance, or who take the steroids to improve libido

- Individuals aiming to improve their physique to perform better in occupations such as bouncing, protection services and the entertainment industry
- Professional and semiprofessional sports people who wish to improve their performance.[2,3,14]

Users come from a wide range of social backgrounds and occupations. Studies have reported AAS use by a diplomat, doctor, hairdresser, manual labourer, fruit-seller, fitness instructor,[2] prison officer, fire fighter, civil engineer, laboratory technician, mechanic, security guard, railway worker, rugby player, nurse, and a PE teacher.[3]
Studies have indicated that:

- Users first try AAS in their early 20s – the youngest age of first use was 15 and the oldest 49, and the mean age of first time use was 21 years.[3]
- Regular use starts during their mid-20s for both men and women.[2]
- One study found the majority of users (64%) to be aged between 20 and 29,[14] and another found them to be between 25 and 39.[15]
- The majority of users (64%) have used AAS for between 1 and 5 years – 21% had used them for less than one year, and a substantial proportion (15%) had taken them for between 6 and 12 years.[14] The longest period of AAS use was for over 20 years.[15]

Adolescents and AAS

AAS use among teenagers has been studied more widely in the USA,[16-18] where the prevalence of use has generally been estimated to be between 5% and 11%. The Canadian Centre for Drug Free Sports study on AAS use among 16 000 11–18-year-olds found that 2.8% had taken them and, based on this, they estimated that 83 000 youngsters in Canada may have taken AAS.[19] In the only British study, Williamson[20] surveyed 687 students at a college of technology on the west coast of Scotland, and found that 4.4% of the males and 1% of the females had taken AAS at some point.

American studies have shown that the more frequently the adolescents studied used AAS, the more frequently they were found to have also used one or more other drugs, such as cocaine, marijuana, and smokeless tobacco.[21] It has thus been concluded that AAS use may be associated with other high-risk behaviours, and that it is part of a "risk-taking syndrome" rather than an isolated behaviour.[22]

Surveys have shown that AAS use is more often associated with "body culture" than with sport.[19] Young people often incorrectly believe that AAS can increase final height.[23] AAS have many positive effects, such as increased self-confidence, increased standing among peers owing to improved musculature, a feeling of wellbeing, and increased libido. These factors may encourage continued use.

Prevalence of AAS use

Precise figures for those using AAS are not available, but estimates can be made from studies and interviews of gym users, surveys of GPs, and statistics available from needle exchange services.

Studies of gymnasium users

Few studies investigating the prevalence of AAS use have been conducted in Britain as a whole. However, useful information has been obtained from several small-scale studies from a single site or urban area, and from anecdotal reports (Table 4.1). Indirect evidence may be gained from the few interview studies of AAS.[14,24] Typically, the studies available have not validated self-reported AAS use by, for example, urine analysis or by repeatability testing, thus weakening the gained evidence.

Table 4.1   Surveys of gymnasium users

Area covered in study	No. of respondents (response rate)	Gym users admitting to AAS use	Study
England and Scotland	1310 men 349 women (59%)	9.1% 2.3%	Korkia and Stimson[2]
West Scotland	41 elite bodybuilders (not stated)	19.5%	McKillop[25]
Northwest England	1105 (58%)	50% at "hardcore" gyms 13% at "fitness" gyms (no free weights) 31% at "mixed" gyms	Lenehan et al.[3]
West Glamorgan	160 (53.3%)	39%	Perry et al.[26]

It is of concern that the Northwest study, which also included interviews with 386 AAS users, found that one in three had started taking AAS in their teens.[3] The authors projected that every 1 in 50 25–29-year-olds in the Northwest may be taking AAS.

After the publication of the Department of Health report, Charles Walker, Head of Sports in the Council of Europe, estimated that in a city the size of London "there will be at least 30 000 and probably as many as 60 000 regular users of anabolic steroids".[27] From observations reported by Williamson,[28] one may expect that out of 200 members in a *typical* gymnasium, 40 will attend regularly and at least 10 will be taking AAS.

It is difficult, on the basis of available data, to estimate the true numbers of AAS users in the whole of Britain. Studies such as the Northwest survey are needed to gauge the true extent of the problem among gymnasium users on a regional basis. The survey findings are not strictly generalisable beyond gymnasium users. For greater ability to generalise to the UK population, further studies are needed of other population groups (Buchan I, personal communication 2001). The available data, however, clearly demonstrate that AAS are used on a nationwide basis, and that it is not a local phenomenon affecting large industrial cities alone.

Needle exchange services

Another indicator of the popularity of AAS use comes from service providers. Needle exchange services (NXS) typically hand out free injecting equipment, provide advice on safe injecting and basic information about drugs, and several offer some basic health screening and advice or consultation with a medical practitioner. A large number of NXS provide this service to AAS users in response to increasing demand, and a dozen specific clinics have been set up specifically for AAS users ("well-steroid user" clinics). At times this provision has been criticised, mainly on grounds of variability in the quality of service offered.[29–31]

Surveys conducted in 1992 showed that in the previous year, 59% of the 88 NXS questioned had served AAS injectors.[2] A few years later, Bellis[32] reported increasing trends in AAS users attending NXS in the Merseyside area: 87 AAS users were recorded in 1991, rising to 546 in 1995. In 1995, AAS were the second most commonly injected drug encountered by services in the Liverpool area,[33] and local indicators suggest that there has been no change in this trend.[34]

Although NXS are widely used, it is clear from talking to NXS staff and users themselves that AAS users do not see themselves as "drug users" and do not feel that they have a "drug problem". A current survey of 115 NXS shows that, of the 63 that replied, 54 had served AAS users in the year 1999. Nine of the respondents had not seen AAS users, or were not sure whether they had served them. Out of the 45 non-respondents at least eight were known by the researchers to be serving AAS users on a regular basis. The number of AAS users served by the agencies varied from a few individuals up to more than 500 in one NXS. Eight services had seen >100 AAS-using clients, four had seen >50, 17 had seen >10, and 10 had seen <10 AAS users in 1999. Of the nine respondents who had not seen AAS users in 1999, two did not know whether they had actually served them, and seven had not served any. Of these seven, two reported that AAS users visited another local NXS.[35] Unfortunately, little is known about the true extent of AAS users accessing NXS and the numbers involved, because the Regional Drug Misuse Databases do not collect this information effectively.

GP surveys

GPs tend to be the first point of contact when medical problems arise, and this may be assumed to be true for AAS users. Both the Department of Health study and the Northwest study suggest that GPs are involved in dealing with the users. Korkia and Stimson[2] found that 2% of their 110 interviewees had been prescribed AAS by GPs, 33% had told their GP about the use of AAS, and 36% were receiving medical monitoring. A third of the 386 interviewees of the Northwest study had told their GP that they were taking AAS; 22% ($n = 83$) were receiving regular medical checks: 45 from their GP and the rest privately. Importantly, Lloyd et al.[36] raised the problem of treating subfertility in men who use AAS. This can lead to lengthy and expensive, totally unnecessary investigations, unless the practitioner is made aware of drug use.

A survey of GPs in the Liverpool, Berkshire, and Birmingham areas[1] found that over a third of the 520 responding GPs (42% response rate) had seen AAS users in their surgeries, although only seven had seen female users. Most (73%) had seen fewer than 3 users, whereas 30% had seen 3–5, 5% 6–11 and 1% 12–17 users in the past 12 months. Only 1% had seen large numbers (>18). Of the 196 who had seen AAS users, 103 suspected that their patients had health problems that were associated with AAS use. A similar survey completed in Bedfordshire[37] found that half of the respondents (60% response rate) reported seeing patients they suspected or knew were misusing AAS. Projections from the whole sample would suggest that at least 30% of Bedfordshire GPs have seen AAS users, depending on the experiences of the non-responders.

Because GPs are in a position to provide medically sound advice to AAS users, questions about their confidence in providing information and advice were included in the Lenehan and McVeigh survey.[1] Only 4% of the respondents felt either confident or very confident; less than a third (26%) felt quite confident; over a third (37%) felt either quite unconfident or very unconfident, and the rest did not feel strongly either way.

British Crime Survey 1996 and 2000

Another tool that may be consulted to gain insight into the use of AAS is the British Crime Survey (BCS). The 1996 survey[38] reported that 1% of male and 1% of female arrestees between the ages of 16 and 59 had ever used AAS. Use was highest among males between ages of 20 and 24, at 3%. More recently, the BCS 2000[38a] reported that 1% of all 17–59-year-old arrestees had used AAS in the previous year, and that 5% of 17–25-year-olds had ever taken them. However, the survey does not link any drug to a crime.

The Council of Europe

Drug use in the sport, health, and fitness setting is seen as a Europe-wide public health issue.[39,40] The different nation states have been instructed to formulate a more unified policy on AAS and associated drug use.[41]

Summary

In summary, several ways of assessing the extent of AAS use in the UK have been employed. Without population-based studies, the prevalence of use in the general population cannot be estimated.

Methods of AAS use

AAS are used mainly in injected (oil-based and water-based) and oral forms. Given orally, testosterone has no pharmacological effect because it is quickly degraded by the liver, and so when taken in this form the drug is often modified by 17α-alkylation to slow down its degradation.[42] Because of this, the oral form is more often associated with liver toxicity. In addition, oral forms require more frequent administration than injected versions. Interviews with AAS users have revealed that the majority (>60%) use both injected and oral forms, with fewer women using injections.[2,3] It appears that the type of AAS used may be an important consideration in the progression of a disease, especially when related to the liver.

Anabolic steroids are mostly self-administered, commonly in large doses for each single drug. The majority of users "stack" AAS, that is, ingest two or more different drugs at the same time; some take more than 10 different drugs during the same cycle. Veterinary drugs are also used, the effects of which have never been tested on humans. Comprehensive lists and descriptions of AAS, their effectiveness, and common side effects as reported by users themselves, can be found in Phillips[43] and Wright.[44]

The drugs are generally taken in cycles,[45] which for men often vary from 8 to 12 weeks on AAS, followed by 8 to 12 weeks off AAS. Some users take no breaks, or take "maintenance" breaks (that is, a relatively small dose of AAS for 8 to 12 weeks). "Female" cycles tend to be shorter, often half of those reported by men. "Cycling" AAS attempts to maximise gains while minimising their harmful effects. Evans,[14] for

Table 4.2 Cycle theories.

Name of cycle	Description
Diamond pattern	Start with minimal dose of one or more AAS, increase dose for several weeks, and then decrease for several weeks to ensure that the body's own testosterone production works before AAS use ceases
Inverted pyramid	Start with a maximum dose and then decrease it gradually. Popular with athletes who are likely to be tested
Three-week blitz	Use one drug at a time for three weeks, changing the preparation over a 15-week period
Feminine cycle	Use two drugs at the same time for four weeks, increasing the dose of one drug each week but keeping the dose of the other constant. Take three weeks off. Drop one drug in favour of the other for the first three weeks after the break. Increase the dose of the chosen drug each week. Use only one drug during the remaining two weeks and taper the dose down

example, describes the cycle of a veteran user: they may take a long-acting agent, such as Sustanon (a mix of 30mg of testosterone propionate, 60mg phenylpropionate, 60mg isocaproate, and 100mg decanoate) during the initial weeks. Then Sustanon is substituted by a shorter-acting agent in the mid-cycle to prevent continuous steroid action during off-cycle. AAS causing minimal fluid retention, such as primobolan/stanozolol, are used during pre-competition by body-builders.

Dosages

It is common for AAS to be taken well in excess of recommended therapeutic dosages. By 1956 it had already been suggested[46] that the side effects of AAS are dose related, and it is worrying that because little information is available regarding maximum effective yet relatively safe dosages, AAS are often taken in excessive quantities.

Dosages for a single preparation have been found to reach up to 34 times the medical recommendation. On average, the men took 3.2 (up to 16), and the women took 2.2 (up to 4) different drugs during the same cycle,[2] which may elevate the circulating androgen levels quite excessively. Some of the users generally do not know the quantity of active ingredients contained in the specific drugs they take: many describe them as "shots", "vials", or "tablets", instead of stating the amount in milligrams. Many AAS come in different strengths, and the lack of knowledge regarding dosages may lead to over (or under) dosing. Millar[47,48] has treated AAS users for the past 15 years in Australia and he has demonstrated that AAS can be administered in far lower doses than currently used by strength athletes, with good gains and no particular side effects. He has been prescribing no more than 500mg/week for up to nine weeks. In one survey of 100 users, 50% were found to take more than 500mg and 12% more than 1000mg of AAS per week, with maximum doses up to 3 200mg weekly.[14]

Polydrug use

Polypharmacy is common among AAS users. A variety of AAS and other drugs are stacked to enhance the effects of AAS or to prevent their unwanted effects. "Non-competitive" users often mimic the AAS and other drug-taking regimens of "competitive" bodybuilders.

As an example, a range of drugs commonly used in conjunction with AAS is detailed in Table 4.3. Although all drugs listed will not be used at the same time, it is common to use one under most classes presented. This table is not a comprehensive list of other drugs AAS users may take, but aims to illustrate their polydrug use.

Table 4.3   Drugs commonly used with AAS

Drug group	Example
Diuretics	Spironalactone and frusemide are commonly used to counteract fluid retention and to promote extreme muscle definition during bodybuilding competitions ('ripped' look)
Insulins	Short- and long-acting insulins to promote glucose uptake by tissues
Thyroid hormones	T_3 and T_4 products and Triacana to accelerate fat metabolism
Spredding agents	Thiomucase (injection, oral, or ointment forms) to "spot" reduce fat (it dehydrates fat cells)
Antioestrogens	Nolvadex (tamoxifen citrate) to prevent gynaecomastia in men and female fat distribution in women
Hypnotics	Triazolam (Halicom) to promote sleep
Opiates	Nubain (nalbuphine hydrochloride) to alleviate training-related pain in muscles and joints (is also highly addictive)
Anticatabolic agents	Aminoglutethimide (Cytodren)
Local steroids	Esiclene and Caverject (alprostadil) irritate the injected site, thereby enhancing muscle definition
Miscellaneous	Reports of the use of the following drugs are also common: antibiotics to combat acne; corticosteroids to treat inflammation; erythropoietin, which some believe will give their veins a "fuller" look, and also to improve workouts through increased oxygen delivery; ephedrine to promote fat loss

Note that the reasons given by athletes for using particular drugs do not necessarily conform to their therapeutic purpose.

As AAS are not used by themselves, but with a number of other drugs and supplements, the evaluation of their efficacy and that of adverse effects is complicated. Later studies have confirmed that the "staple" of drugs has generally not changed much since the Korkia and Stimson report.[2] Regional variations in the supply of drugs is generally believed to influence the patterns of use.

Growth hormone, insulin, and insulin-like growth factor-1 use

The use of growth hormone (GH) is estimated to be high in both bodybuilding and sport, despite its high cost of approximately £400 per monthly course of 2IU/day.[14] Insulin-like growth factor-1 (IGF-1) is also expensive, at approximately £600 per milligram. Regimens vary and some users take 30 micrograms per day for a month, or 50 micrograms on training days for a month.[24] Some users believe that GH increases muscle size and strength without the side effects caused by AAS, but anecdotal reports of their effectiveness have remained controversial. The combined use of AAS and GH may prove to be a major cardiovascular risk in future years when the high-dose/long-term users reach a more advanced age.

Growth hormone is often taken together with insulin because of their synergistic effect. The release of somatomedins, such as IGF-1, is achieved by GH administration. IGF-1 emerged on the US "black market" in the early 1990s and spread to the UK just before the mid-1990s. Parry[24] interviewed 189 male bodybuilders and weightlifters to explore their IGF-1 use, and found that 14% had taken it. IGF-1 is taken with GH and AAS because it appears to work more effectively in a high androgenic environment. Parry[24] found the attitude of the 67% who had not yet used IGF-1 worrying, because despite not knowing any facts about the drug, all were prepared to try it. Again, anecdotal reports of its efficacy in increasing size and strength are controversial. The controversy with GH and IGF-1 may be the result of individual responsiveness, dose, or the actual drug content (or lack of it) when bought from the "black market".

Recreational drug use

In addition to "medicinal" drug use, social drugs are also taken in conjunction with AAS: Korkia and Stimson[2] reported that of the 110 AAS users they interviewed, 81% had consumed alcohol, 18% amfetamines, 24% cannabis, 30% tobacco, 4% cocaine, and 5% other drugs, such as ecstasy and LSD. Morrison[49] interviewed AAS and cocaine users via outreach services and suggested that the combined use of the two may be widespread. In response to pressure to maintain size and appearance and to remain competitive on the job market, older doormen may use cocaine along with AAS to train, while others take it to stay awake during night shifts. According to users, cocaine allows 25 minutes of extreme-load training, exceeding any normal capacity to push the weights. Training in this state is commonly referred to as totally manic–psychotic, and possibly a danger to others around the user when/if emotions ride high. The effects of a dose of cocaine for training purposes last for about 45 minutes. The cardiovascular dangers of combined use of AAS and cocaine in an already compromised heart were highlighted in this report and in animal studies.[50]

Nubain

Nalbuphine hydrochloride (Nubain) is an opioid-based parenteral analgesic. Increasing reports of its use in sport have appeared since the mid-1990s, mainly to relieve and to mask pain from injury and training-related muscle soreness. AAS users also take it to calm down before a competition and for its stress-reducing anticatabolic actions.[14,34,51] For example, Evans[14] found that 6 out of 100 users had taken Nubain. Dependence has been reported in AAS users in the British and American medical literature,[51,52] coupled with numerous anecdotal reports of severe withdrawal problems and dependence from needle exchange service workers.[35] Wines et al.[52] found high rates of psychotic symptoms and medical complications in the 11 AAS/Nubain users they interviewed.

Summary of polydrug use

The use of AAS and a multitude of other drugs, including recreational/illicit drugs, may lead to unpredictable consequences. The assessment of health risks involved in AAS use must always take account of all other drugs that may be consumed. Those who take a number of different types of preparations in high dosages can expect to experience a range of side effects. The use of various psychostimulants and AAS together may increase the likelihood of harm to self and others.

Adverse effects of AAS

The adverse effects of AAS were discussed in detail in Chapter 3. The methodologies of a number of studies of the possible adverse effects of AAS have been questioned. Many have small sample sizes, lack control groups, fail to confirm exposure to AAS (for example by urinalysis), fail to consider the veracity of self-reports, and fail to consider possible confounders, such as other drug use (Buchan I, personal communication 2001). Acceptable evidence exists for androgen-sensitive liver neoplasia, gynaecomastia, dependence, and increase in risk behaviours for sexually transmitted infections. The major gap in the evidence is a lack of long-term prospective studies of the effect of AAS use in non-athletes, especially with regard to cardiovascular risks.

Common signs of anabolic steroid use

The actions of AAS and the reasons for their use were discussed in the previous chapter. Common signs of use include:

- Skin: acne, needle marks in large muscle groups, body hair in women, bruising with minor injuries
- Face: facial hair in women, puffiness caused by fluid retention
- Chest: gynaecomastia in men and atrophied breasts in women
- Genital: testicular atrophy in men and clitoral enlargement in women, infertility
- Musculoskeletal: marked muscle hypertrophy, disproportionate development of the neck, shoulders, and chest
- Other: insomnia, lack of concentration, mood swings, depression, deepened voice in women.

Financial costs

Using AAS is very expensive. The average cost of a "cycle" was reported to be about £70 (£13–£500) by Korkia and Stimson[2] and £140 (£15–£2000) by Lenehan et al.[3] Bodybuilders and weightlifters from 14 different gyms in London and the Bournemouth area reported spending between £500 and £2500 annually on performance-enhancing drugs, amounting to 45% of the total cost of training.[24] Evans'[14] interviewees spent between £40 and £370 per a typical four-week period on AAS.

Availability of AAS

Anabolic steroids are easily available through gyms, the internet, and mail order. Friends appear to have an important role in introducing individuals to AAS and as sources of information. Interviews with AAS users suggest that it is easy to get them, though they do not always get exactly the drugs they wanted.[2] In 1993, friends were frequently involved in supplying AAS to each other.

Although the possession of AAS with intent to supply/share was made illegal in the UK in 1996, the enforcement agencies are not trying to catch and prosecute users. However, they have powers to stop and prosecute dealers.[53] As a consequence of legislative changes, the supply of AAS now appears to be almost exclusively in the hands of dealers. Hence AAS users may come into contact with other illicit drugs. Gym owners now seldom deal in them, fearing the loss of livelihood.[54,55] Studies from the USA consistently demonstrate that AAS use and the use of other illicit drugs are heavily correlated,[21,22,56] and for this reason the new legislation may result in more harm and less protection. The contents, quality, cleanliness, and general safety of "black market" products have been shown to be compromised, and cases of poisoning, infection, and mental illness have been reported.[57]

Dangers of the "black market"

Ritsch and Musshoff[58] evaluated 40 AAS obtained from the German "black market" and found that 37.5% of the drugs contained different or none of the pharmacological compounds labelled. In Merseyside, McVeigh and Lenehan[59] had four AAS tested. Although all contained some AAS, they varied from 43% to 73% of their stated content. In response to concerns about the prevalence and dangers of counterfeit AAS, the Welsh Office funded a study that enabled the purchase and analysis of "black market" products.[60] Again, a vast discrepancy between actual and labelled ingredients was found: 4 different brands of nandrolone, 0–157% of stated active drug content; 3 brands of methandienone, 85–169%; 4 brands of stanozolol, 73–111%; and 4 samples of testosterone, 59–102%. The investigator highlighted several key issues:

- The danger of overdosing – especially relevant for women who strive to avoid the androgenic effects of the drug
- The questionable sterility of injectable drugs (there were reports of sunflower cooking oil having been used instead of arachis oil)
- Two samples of the same drug from the same "manufacturer" contained differing amounts of AAS.

An extreme case of the dangers of the "black market" supply is described by Perry and Hughes:[57] a 30-year-old AAS user had acquired haldol decanoate from the "black market" in the belief that it was the commonly used AAS nandrolone decanoate. He developed acute depression and suicidal ideas, and continued to have psychiatric problems for at least nine months.

A further problem with "black market" supply of AAS is that the distribution network itself may act as a gateway to trying out other drugs to which the AAS user would not otherwise be exposed.

Sources of information about AAS

Friendship networks play a key role in getting into training and taking AAS, and tend to be the main source of information for most users, followed by underground handbooks and dealers.[2,3] It is of concern that those who sell the drugs also provide much of the information about drug combinations, "effective" dosages, cycle lengths, and possible side effects. In the absence of reliable medical and scientific information, AAS use is largely based on the trial and error results of other users. "Underground" handbooks often contain information that is inaccurate.

Also, drug availability from the dealer tends to be an important consideration. The unsuitable advice given by men to women users has been highlighted.[59,61] Many NXS provide leaflets and some have a specialist service for AAS users; however, the majority of this service provision involves supplying sterile injecting equipment. Agencies such as NXS, that deal with large numbers of users, often have no specific training and/or information point to turn to for consultation, therefore information provided may at times be unreliable. Furthermore, the surveys of GPs in the north and south of England suggest that they are, on the whole, not confident about advising AAS users. Medical checks for users of AAS are not widely available, and this lack of access to appropriate medical advice has not helped in curtailing irresponsible drug regimens.[48]

Interventions to prevent AAS use or minimise harm

Educating AAS users about the possible adverse effects of steroids may be difficult, as 44% of the interviewees in the Korkia and Stimson study[2] said that they would continue using AAS even if it was shown that they do cause life-threatening conditions, such as cancer. Interventions to prevent the use of AAS or to minimise their harm may be primary, secondary, or tertiary.

- Primary interventions aim to prevent AAS use in those who have never used them.

- Secondary interventions aim to prevent use in non-dependent users.
- Tertiary interventions aim to prevent or limit use in dependent users, or to treat adverse effects in AAS users.

The majority of studies into primary (and secondary) prevention have been conducted in American high schools with members of football teams. Interventions comprised solely of fact-based education have been found to significantly increase the participants' knowledge of AAS, but have not been found to significantly change attitudes towards AAS, or intentions to use them.[62] Even a fact-based intervention which emphasised the negative effects of AAS showed the same general results but, surprisingly, there was a significant increase in the desire to use AAS.[63] Only when the intervention approach is more comprehensive, with fact-based education being supplemented with refusal skills role play, peer-led sessions, and integration with a strength training programme, are significant decreases in self-reported use, desire to use, and intention to use observed. This effect was maintained at one year post intervention AAS.[64,65]

In terms of tertiary prevention, two studies had clearly defined experimental methods for assessing the effectiveness of measures to prevent harm due to AAS in established users. One intervention was a problem-oriented treatment programme.[66] From an initial 15 AAS users, five were lost to follow up, eight stopped using AAS, and two halved their drug intake. Follow-up was for three to eight months. Despite the seeming success of this intervention, it is noted that the evidence is weak because of the small numbers and lack of a control group.

The second intervention was a physician-controlled prescription programme that involved medical assessments prior to prescribing AAS, and repeat prescription dependent upon medical monitoring and patient education.[47] Each of the 169 participants was followed up for between three and five years. It was observed that adverse effects of AAS were minimal, and speculated that less AAS was used than would be expected without physician-controlled prescription. However, as with the other study, the evidence is weak owing to lack of a control group.

Further research should build on the foundations of these studies, as after identifying that there are a significant number of non-competitive athletes using AAS, and that there are potential adverse health effects, efforts should be concentrated on both preventing individuals from starting AAS use and minimising harm to those who insist on continued use.

Summary

This chapter has highlighted the growing problem of AAS use among those not involved in competitive sports. New users are generally in their early 20s when they commence AAS use, take dosages and drug combinations that are not advised, and may obtain them from dubious sources. Emphasis must be placed on educating users, and also medical practitioners who may be consulted in the event of difficulties encountered by users. This education of medical practitioners may take place at both the undergraduate and the postgraduate level. Consideration should be given to including the subject of doping in the undergraduate medical curriculum, as part of any training received by doctors about drug abuse in the core curricular themes "The individual in society" and "Personal and professional development". Training in drug misuse in sport should form part of postgraduate medical education for any doctor likely to come into contact with such drug misusers in their work, and should also be an essential element of any programme or course on sports medicine.

References

1 Lenehan P, McVeigh J. General Practitioner questionnaire survey. *The Drugs and Sport Information Service*, Liverpool, 1996. (Unpublished.)

2 Korkia PK, Stimson GV. *Anabolic Steroid Use in Great Britain: an exploratory investigation*. The Centre for Research on Drugs and Health Behaviour. A report for the Department of Health, the Welsh Office and the Chief Scientist Office. Scottish Home and Health Department, 1993.

3 Lenehan P, Bellis M, McVeigh J. Anabolic steroid use in the North West of England. *J Performance Enhancing Drugs* 1996;1: 57–70.

4 Boje O. Doping. *Bull Health Org League of Nations* 1939;8: 439–69.

5 Boone JB, Lambert CP, Flynn MG, Michaud TJ, Rodriguez-Zayas JA, Andres FF. Resistance exercise effects on plasma cortisol, testosterone and creatinine kinase activity in anabolic-androgenic steroid users. *Int J Sports Med* 1990;11: 293–7.

6 Sheffield-Moore M. Androgens and the control of skeletal muscle protein synthesis. *Ann Med* 2000;32: 181–6.

7 Demling RH, Orgill DP. The anticatabolic and wound healing effects of testosterone analog oxandrolone after severe burn injury. *J Crit Care* 2000;15: 12–17.

8 Itl T. Neurophysiological effects of hormones in humans: computer EEG profiles of sex and hypothalamic hormones. In: Schar EJ, ed. *Hormones, Behaviour and Psychopathology*. New York: Raven Press, 1976.

9 Rubinow DR, Schmidt PJ. Androgens, brain and behaviour. *Am J Psychiatry* 1996;**153**: 974–84.

10 Haupt H, Rovere G. Anabolic steroids: A review of the literature. *Am J Sports Med* 1984;**12**: 469–84.

11 Lamb DR. Anabolic steroids in athletics: How well do they work and how dangerous are they? *Am J Sports Med* 1984;**12**: 31–8.

12 Yesalis CE, Streit AL, Vicary JR, Friedl KE, Brannon D, Buckley W. Anabolic steroid use: Indications of habituation among adolescents. *J Drug Educ* 1989;**19**: 103–16.

13 Rasmussen BB, Volpi E, Gore DC, Wolfe RR. Androstenedione does not stimulate muscle protein anabolism in young healthy men. *J Clin Endocrinol Metab* 2000;**85**: 55–9.

14 Evans NA. Gym and tonic: A profile of 100 male steroid users. *Br J Sports Med* 1997;**31**: 54–8.

15 Pates R, Barry C. Steroid use in Cardiff: A problem for whom? *J Performance Enhancing Drugs* 1996;**1**: 92–7.

16 Dezelsky T, Toohey J, Shaw R. Non-medical drug use behaviour at five United States universities: a 15-year study. *Bull Narcotics* 1985;**37**: 49–53.

17 Buckley W, Yesalis C, Friedl K, Anderson W, Streit A, Wright J. Estimated prevalence of anabolic steroid use among male high school seniors. *JAMA* 1988;**260**: 3441–5.

18 Johnson MD, Jay MS, Shoup B, Rickert VI. Anabolic steroid use by male adolescents. *Pediatrics* 1989;**83**: 921–4.

19 Melia P. Sports for all! But is it suitable for children? *Int J Drug Policy* 1994;**5**: 34–9.

20 Williamson DJ. Misuse of anabolic drugs. *BMJ* 1993;**306**: 61.

21 DuRant RH, Rickert VI, Ashworth CS, Newman C, Slavens G. Use of multiple drugs among adolescents who use anabolic steroids. *N Engl J Med* 1993;**328**: 922–6.

22 Middleman AB, Faulkner AH, Woods ER, Emans SJ, DuRant RH. High-risk behaviours among high-school students in Massachusetts who use anabolic steroids. *Pediatrics* 1995;**96**: 268–72.

23 Tanner SM, Miller DW, Alongi C. Anabolic steroid use by adolescents: prevalence, motives, and knowledge of risks. *Clin J Sport Med* 1995;**5**: 108–15.

24 Parry DA. Insulin-like growth factor-1 (IGF-1). A new generation of performance enhancement by athletes. *J Performance Enhancing Drugs* 1996;**1**: 48–51.

25 McKillop G. Drug abuse in bodybuilders in the West of Scotland. *Scot Med J* 1987;**32**: 39–41.

26 Perry HM, Wright D, Littlepage BNC. Dying to be big: a review of anabolic steroid use. *Br J Sports Med* 1992;**26**: 259–61.

27 Walker G. Conference Proceedings: *The 4th Permanent World Conference on Anti-doping in Sport,* 5–8 September 1993, The Sports Council (UK), 1994.

28 Williamson DJ. Edinburgh's lesser known drug problems. *Edinburgh Med* 1991;**65**: 6–7.

29 Morrison CM. The cost of running a well steroid user service. *Relay* 1995;**1**: 10–11.

30 Williamson K, Davis M, McBride A. A well-steroid user clinic. *Druglink* 1992;Sept/Oct,15.
31 Perry HM. The pitfalls of a well steroid user clinic. *Relay* 1994;1: 5.
32 Bellis D. Prevalence and patterns of anabolic steroid use. *The 3rd Annual Conference of The Drugs and Sport Information Service* Liverpool, 2 July 1996.
33 Lenehan P, McVeigh J. Anabolic steroid use in Liverpool. *The Drugs and Sport Information Service,* Liverpool, 1996. (Unpublished.)
34 Lenehan P. Director of the Drugs and Sport Information Service, Liverpool, *personal communications,* 2000.
35 Korkia P, Lenehan P. Numbers of anabolic steroid injectors visiting needle exchange agencies in England and Wales. (Unpublished.)
36 Lloyd FH, Powell P, Murdoch AP. Anabolic steroid abuse by bodybuilders and male subfertility. *BMJ* 1996;**313**: 100–1.
37 Korkia P. Anabolic steroid use: A Survey of General Practitioners in the South of England. [Abstract]. *Proceedings of the 2nd European Congress of Sport and Exercise Science,* Copenhagen, August 1997.
38 British Crime Survey. London: Home Office, 1996.
38a British Crime Survey. HO Research Series 205. London: Home Office, 2000.
39 Council of Europe (Griffiths P, Bacchus L). *Use of Anabolic Steroids and other Doping Substances outside Competitive Sport: Literature review and European key informant survey.* Strasbourg: Council of Europe, 1998.
40 Council of Europe (Shaphiro H). Public Health Committee. Committee of experts on pharmaceutical questions. *The non-sport use of prohibited anabolic and androgenic substances: clinical aspects.* Strasbourg: Council of Europe, 1998.
41 Council of Europe, Strasbourg, 7 July 1999. Committee for the Development of Sport, Anti-Doping Convention, *Sprint Seminar on non-sport use of banned substances.* Lisbon, Conclusions.
42 Wadler G, Hainline H. Anabolic Steroids. In: Ryan A, ed. *Drugs and the Athlete. Contemporary Exercise and Sports Medicine Series.* Philadelphia: FA Davis Company, 1989.
43 Phillips WN. *Anabolic Reference Guide.* USA: Mile High Publishing, 1991.
44 Wright JE. *Anabolic Steroids and Sports Vol II.* USA: Sports Science Consultants, 1992.
45 Duchaine D. *The underground steroid handbook II.* Venice, CA: HLR Technical Books, 1989.
46 Kochakian CD, Endahl BR. Changes in body weight in normal and castrated rats by different doses of testosterone propionate. *Proc Soc Exp Biol Med* 1959;**100**: 520–22.
47 Millar AP. Licit steroid use: hope for the future. *Br J Sports Med* 1994;**28**: 79–83.
48 Millar AP. Anabolic steroids: A personal pilgrimage. *J Performance Enhancing Drugs* 1996;1: 4–9.
49 Morrison CM. Cocaine misuse in anabolic steroid users. *J Performance Enhancing Drugs* 1996;1: 10–15.
50 Phillis BD, Irvine RJ, Kennedy JA. Combined cardiac effects of cocaine and anabolic steroid, nandrolone, in the rat. *Eur J Pharmacol* 2000;**398**: 263–72.

51 McBride AJ, Williamson K, Petersen T. Three cases of nalbuphine hydrochloride dependence associated with anabolic steroid use. *Br J Sports Med* 1996;**30**: 69–70.
52 Wines DJ Jr, Gruber AJ, Pope HG Jr, Lukas SE. Nalbuphine hydrochloride dependence in anabolic steroid users. *Am J Addiction* 1999;**8**: 161–4.
53 Morgan I. Anabolic steroid legislation. *J Performance Enhancing Drugs* 1996;**1**: 52–3.
54 Lowther J. The new law and reclassification of anabolic steroids. A personal view. *J Performance Enhancing Drugs* 1996;**1**: 54–6.
55 Kayes K. Anabolic steroids and control strategies. *The 3rd Annual Conference of The Drugs and Sport Information Service*, Liverpool: 2 July 1996.
56 Yesalis CE, Kennedy NJ, Kopstein AN, Bahrke MS. Anabolic-androgenic steroid use in the United States. *JAMA* 1993;**270**: 1217–21.
57 Perry HM, Hughes GW. A case of affective disorder associated with the misuse of "anabolic steroid". *Br J Sports Med* 1992;**26**: 219–20.
58 Ritsch M, Musshoff F. Dangers and risks of "black market" anabolic steroid abuse in sports – gas chromatography–mass spectrometry analyses. *Sportverletz Sportschaden* 2000;**14**: 1–11.
59 McVeigh J, Lenehan P. Counterfeits and fakes. *Relay* 1994;**1**: 8–9.
60 Perry H. Counterfeit: Fake anabolic steroids and hazards of their use. *Relay* 1995;**1**: 9–11.
61 Korkia P, Lenehan P, McVeigh J. Non-medical use of androgens among women. *J Performance Enhancing Drugs* 1996;**1**: 71–6.
62 Goldberg L, Bosworth E, Bents RT, Trevisan L. Effect of an anabolic steroid education program on knowledge and attitudes of high school football players. *J Adolesc Health Care* 1990;**11**: 210–14.
63 Goldberg L, Bents R, Bosworth E, Trevisan L, Elliot DL. Anabolic education and adolescents: do scare tactics work? *Pediatrics* 1991;**87**: 283–6.
64 Goldberg L, Elliot D, Clarke GN *et al*. Effects of a multidimensional anabolic steroid prevention intervention. The adolescents training and learning to avoid steroids (ATLAS) program. *JAMA* 1996;**276**: 1555–62.
65 Goldberg L, MacKinnon DP, Elliot DL, Moe EL, Clarke G, Cheong J. The adolescents training and learning to avoid steroids program: Preventing drug use and promoting health behaviours. *Arch Pediatr Adolesc Med* 2000;**154**: 332–8.
66 Frankle MA, Leffers D. Athletes on anabolic-androgenic steroids: New approach diminishes health problems. *Phys Sports Med* 1992;**20**: 75–87.

5: Doping in elite-level sport

The extent of doping in elite-level sport

It is difficult to arrive at a precise estimate of the prevalence of doping in elite sport, as those involved in the practice will normally seek to conceal their activities. However, the available evidence suggests that the use of performance-enhancing drugs has increased substantially since doping controls were introduced in the 1960s, and that the use of drugs in elite-level sport is now widespread.

It is generally agreed that the modern increase in the use of performance-enhancing drugs dates from the late 1950s and early 1960s. By 1968, an estimated one third of the United States track and field team had used steroids at the pre-Olympic training camp.[1] By the mid-1970s performance-enhancing drugs had already come to be regarded as an essential aid to training and/or competition by many athletes,[2] and there is some evidence to suggest that since then their use has become even more widespread.

In her evidence to the US Senate Judiciary Committee Hearing on Steroid Abuse in America, chaired in April 1989 by Senator Joseph Biden Jr, Pat Connolly, a coach of the US women's track and field team, estimated that, of the 50 members of the team at the 1984 Olympics, "probably 15 of them had used steroids. Some of them were medallists". Asked by Senator Biden whether the number of athletes using steroids had increased by the time of the Seoul Olympics of 1988, Connolly replied, "Oh, yes. Oh, yes, it went up a lot". She estimated that "At least 40% of the women's team in Seoul had probably used steroids at some time in their preparation for the Games" (cited in Dubin[3]).

Shortly before the US Senate Judiciary Committee Hearing, the Australian government, concerned about the apparently increasing use of banned substances by athletes, referred the issue to a Senate standing committee for investigation and report. The committee heard evidence that approximately 70% of Australian athletes who competed internationally had taken drugs, and that one quarter of the Australian track and field team at the Seoul Olympics had used drugs. The committee accepted that "drug taking in Australian sport is widespread, and that anabolic steroids in particular are used in any sport in which power is an advantage". They also concluded that "drugs are being used at all levels of sport and by most age groups, although the extent of drug use varies widely from one sport to another".[4]

The most systematic and reliable evidence on the extent of doping in elite sport is that which was presented to the Dubin Commission of Inquiry in Canada. Dubin took evidence from no fewer than 46 Canadian athletes who had used anabolic steroids, and he concluded:

After hearing evidence and meeting with knowledgeable people from Canada, the United States, Australia, New Zealand, and elsewhere, I am convinced that the problem is widespread not only in Canada but also around the world. The evidence shows that banned performance-enhancing substances and, in particular, anabolic steroids are being used by athletes in almost every sport, most extensively in weight lifting and track and field.[3]

There is no evidence to suggest that the problem has lessened in the last few years. Anthony Millar, Research Director at the Institute of Sports Medicine in Sydney, Australia, wrote in 1996 of an "epidemic of drug usage" in sport, and suggested that the use of performance-enhancing drugs "is widespread and growing, not only in the athletic community, but also among recreational athletes".[5] In a survey of 448 British Olympic athletes carried out in 1995, 48% felt that drug use was a problem in international competition in their sport (in track and field the figure was 86%). Nor did these elite British athletes feel that the problem was being tackled effectively by the existing system of doping controls: 23% of athletes felt that drug use had increased over the previous 12 months, compared to just 6% who felt it had decreased.[6] More recently, the revelations about doping in the 1998 Tour de France provided unambiguous evidence that doping in professional cycling is both widespread and systematically organised.[7] It is also clear that drugs are widely used in other sport-related contexts. In a British survey of anabolic steroid use in "hardcore" gyms (defined as gyms having predominantly heavy weight-training equipment, competitive bodybuilders, and relatively few female members), over 29% of gym users were currently using anabolic steroids.[8] This was discussed in more detail in Chapter 4.

Houlihan[9] has noted that the objectives of current anti-doping policy are not clearly defined, and that the "techniques for measuring progress towards policy objectives are poor, relying mainly on trends in the number of positive test results". It might be noted that both the International Olympic Committee and, at home, UK Sport, use the number of positive tests as an indication of such progress. However, the Dubin Commission pointed out that the incidence of positive test results is a poor index – some would argue so poor as to be virtually worthless – of the extent of drug use by athletes. Initial findings from the European Commission's Doping in Sport Project do indeed suggest that drug abuse is more widespread than official figures show. The conclusions of this study will be used to formulate a pan-European anti-doping awareness campaign.[10] Overall, there is clearly a pressing need to define more clearly the objectives of anti-doping policy, and to specify more clearly the criteria for monitoring the success of that policy.

Reasons for the increasing use of drugs in sport

The medicalisation of sport

Two key social processes provide the essential context for understanding the increase in the use of performance-enhancing drugs in sport since the second world war. These are:

- Improvements in chemical technology: the so-called "pharmacological revolution" which developed from the 1950s and 1960s resulted in the development of more potent, more selective, and less toxic drugs.
- The growing involvement of physicians in the medical management of athletes.

These two processes are central to what has been described as the medicalisation of sport, which is an aspect of the medicalisation of society more generally.[7]

The medicalisation process in society has involved growing dependence on professionally provided care, dependence on drugs to cure all ills, both physical and psychological, the medicalisation of prevention, and increased expectations of lay people. The use of drugs in sport must be viewed in this context. In recent years the medicalisation process has enveloped sport: it would be unrealistic to expect athletes to insulate themselves from our increasingly pill-dependent culture.[9] Central to this has been the development, particularly since the 1960s, of sports medicine, which is based on the idea that the highly trained athlete has special medical needs and therefore requires special medical supervision.

A culture has evolved which encourages the treatment not just of injured athletes, but also of healthy athletes, with drugs. For example, Voy,[11] former chief medical officer for the US Olympic Committee, recorded the daily intake of legal drugs of a national track star: vitamin E, 160mg; B-complex capsules, four times per day; vitamin C, 2000mg; vitamin B_6, 150mg; calcium tablets, four times per day; magnesium tablets, twice a day; zinc tablets, three times a day; royal jelly capsules; garlic tablets; cayenne tablets; eight aminos; γ-Oryzanol; Mega Vit Pack; supercharge herbs; dibencozide; glandular tissue complex; natural steroid complex; inosine; orchid testicle extract; pyridium; ampicillin; and hair rejuvenation formula with biotin.

Sports medicine is concerned not just with the "prevention, diagnosis, and treatment of exercise related illnesses and injuries", but also with the "maximisation of performance",[12] and as such, goes beyond the treatment of sports injury. Moreover, as the rewards associated with winning have increased, so the role of sports medicine practitioners in maximising performance has become more important. One consequence of this growing concern with the maximisation of performance[13] has been to make top-class athletes more and more dependent on increasingly sophisticated systems of medical support in their efforts to run faster, to jump further, or to compete more effectively in their chosen sport; indeed, at the highest levels the quality of medical support may make the difference between success and failure. Brown and Benner,[14] for example, have pointed out that, as increased importance has been placed on winning, athletes, in order to increase their advantage in competitions, have turned to "mechanical (exercise, massage), nutritional (vitamins, minerals), psychological (discipline, transcendental meditation), and pharmacological (medicines, drugs) methods ... A major emphasis has been placed on the non-medical use of drugs, particularly anabolic steroids, central nervous system stimulants, depressants and analgesics".

In addition, we should not forget that athletes live in a society where there is widespread abuse of drugs, and will also be exposed to drugs in recreational settings.[9,15] The "post-game" party is often an integral component of many sports. Recreational drugs may also be used to cope with the pressures of training and competition.

Pressures faced by athletes

It would, however, be quite wrong to suggest that athletes are simply unwilling "victims" of medical imperialism. A number of developments in the structure of sporting competition, particularly in the post-second world war period, have led sportsmen and women increasingly to turn for help to anyone who can hold out the promise of improving their level of performance. The most important of these developments are probably those that have been associated with the politicisation of sport, particularly at the international level, and those that have been associated with massive increases in the rewards – particularly the material rewards – associated with sporting success. Both these processes have had the consequence of increasing the competitiveness of sport, and one aspect of this increasing competitiveness has been the downgrading, in relative terms, of the traditional value associated with taking part while greatly increasing the value attached to winning.

It is important to note that this trend towards the growing competitiveness of sport not only provides an essential context for understanding doping in sport, but that it has also had a number of other important health-related consequences for sportsmen and women. In particular, the growing competitiveness of sport has had significant health "costs" for athletes, partly because of the increasingly intense training programmes, but also because of the increasing constraints to "play hurt", that is, to continue competing while injured.[16,17]

Donohoe and Johnson[18] have pointed out that to "succeed in modern sport, athletes are forced to train longer, harder, and earlier in life. They may be rewarded by faster times, better performances and increased fitness, but there is a price to pay for such intense training". Part of the price of this and of the readiness to continue training and competing despite injury (often encouraged by coaches) is paid in the form of overuse and recurrent injuries, which now constitute a serious problem in sport, and not just at the adult elite level. As Donohoe and Johnson[18] have noted, the "long-term effects of overuse injuries are not known, but some concerned doctors have asked whether today's gold medallists could be crippled by arthritis by the age of 30", and they cite world-class competitors who have, in their words, "been plagued by a succession of overuse injuries".

Perhaps of even greater concern are the health effects of increasingly intensive training routines on young children. Donnelly[19] highlighted a disturbing trend of parents who encourage their children to become heavily involved in professional sport at an early age because of the possibility of a financially successful career. This trend is further exacerbated by the variety of attempts made to establish schemes for the early identification of athletic talent, and by government and organisations justifying spending on elite participation as a response to increasing demands for international success in sport.

Donnelly notes that injuries characteristic of overtraining among young athletes have been widely reported in the literature. Such injuries were reported by a majority of the recently retired high-level athletes who were interviewed for his own study, and who talked about their own experiences as young athletes. It is therefore important for those responsible for the medical care of child athletes to remind those in charge of their training programmes that the athletes in question are children, that particular care should be taken to ensure that they are not given training schedules appropriate for adults, and that they are not subject to overtraining. Sports Coach UK, the national foundation for coaching, issues a code of conduct which cautions coaches to be aware of the physical needs of athletes, especially those still growing, and to ensure that training loads and intensities are appropriate.[20] Children should also be particularly protected from the use of drugs, as substances that may not damage a fully developed athlete may have serious consequences for a child who is still growing.[21]

The increasing competitiveness of sport

The emphasis that has come to be placed on the importance of winning and which has come to be such a striking feature of modern sports, particularly at the elite level, is a relatively modern phenomenon. Dunning and Sheard,[22] for example, have noted that the amateur ethos which was articulated in late 19th-century England emphasised the importance of sporting activity as "an 'end in itself', ie simply for the pleasure afforded, with a corresponding downgrading of achievement, striving, training and specialisation". The competitive element was important, but the achievement of victory was not supposed to be central; indeed, the English public school elite which articulated the amateur ethos were opposed to cups and leagues because such competitions were, it was held, conducive to an overemphasis on victory and to an "overly serious" attitude to sport which, ideally, should be played for the intrinsic pleasure it provided, rather than for the extrinsic pleasure associated with winning cups or medals.[22] This offers a striking contrast with the highly competitive character of modern sport, and with the much greater emphasis which has in more recent times come to be placed on the importance of winning.

The politicisation of sport

Although the relationship between politics and sport is by no means exclusively a post-second world war phenomenon – witness the "Nazi Olympics" of 1936 – some have argued that sport has become increasingly politicised in the period since 1945. Of particular significance in this respect was the development of communist regimes in many parts of Eastern Europe and, associated with this, the emergence of the Cold War and of superpower rivalry. Within this context, international sporting competition took on a significance going far beyond the bounds of sport itself, for sport – at least within the context of east–west relations – became an extension of the political, military, and economic competition that characterised relationships between the superpowers and their associated blocs.[9,23,24] As the report of the Amateur Athletics Association Drug Abuse enquiry in 1988 pointed out, one factor in the increasing use of drugs "was the decision by a number of countries to regard success in international sport including athletics as ... valuable ... particularly for political and propaganda reasons".[2]

Comparisons of the number of Olympic medals won by the United States and the Soviet Union – or, following the admission of separate teams from West Germany and East Germany from the 1968 Olympics, the medals won by the two Germanies – thus came to be very important, for the winning of medals came to be seen as a symbol not only of national pride but also of the superiority of one political system over another. As many governments came to see international sporting success as an important propaganda weapon in the east–west struggle, so those athletes who emerged as winners came increasingly to be treated as national heroes, with rewards, sometimes provided by national governments, to match.

Franke and Berendonk[25] have described the doping programme in the former GDR, carried out for largely political reasons, as "one of the largest pharmacological experiments in history". Evidence indicates that adolescents were given steroids disguised as vitamin pills, and mestalanone was given to female gymnasts and volleyball players without having been approved for administration to humans in clinical phase I trials.

Sport and commercialisation

The increasing competitiveness of sport has also been associated with its growing commercialisation, particularly in the west. Although the winning of an Olympic medal has undoubtedly always been considered an honour, it is indisputably the case that in recent years the non-honorific rewards, and in particular the financial rewards, associated with Olympic success have increased massively. Voy, for example, has pointed to the huge financial rewards which are available in the United States (and, we might note, increasingly in other western countries) to Olympic gold medal winners, who are able to demand not only very high appearance fees for competing in major meetings but, much more importantly, can also earn huge incomes from sponsorship, from television commercials, and from product endorsement. However, Voy has noted that such fabulous rewards are available only to those who come first, for, as he put it, "second place doesn't count".[26]

Central to the increasing commercialisation of sport have been two processes: the development of sports sponsorship, and the increasing global audience, via television, for both live and recorded sport. A report by the European Group on Ethics[27] concluded that doping in sport is fuelled by a desire for entertainment surpassing all previous limits. As Gratton and Taylor[28] have noted, sports sponsorship "hardly existed as an economic activity before 1970 in Britain, yet by 1999 it was estimated to be worth £350 million". They add that, globally, sports sponsorship is a massive industry estimated to be worth around $20 billion in 1999, having grown by over 300% in the 1990s alone. Significantly, sports sponsorship is now the dominant form of sponsorship, accounting for over two thirds of all sponsorship activity.

In relation to the Olympic movement, it was the 1984 Los Angeles Games which, as the International Olympic Committee has noted, "marked the beginning of the most successful era of corporate sponsorship". In the following year the IOC created The Olympic Programme (TOP) and, over the next 15 years, the TOP programme increased its sponsorship finance sixfold, from US $95 million for TOP I (1985–88) to US $550+ million for TOP IV (1998–2000). The increase in the IOC's revenues from selling television rights to the Games has been even more spectacular. The global television fees for the 1980 Moscow games were US $101 million, increasing to US $287 million for the 1984 Los Angeles Games. The fee has increased substantially at every subsequent summer Olympics, and the estimated fee for the TV rights for the 2004 Athens Olympics is US $1,498 million. Over the same period, the fees for television rights to theWinter Games have increased 35-fold, from US $21 million for the 1980 games at Lake Placid to an estimated US $738 million for the 2002 games at Salt Lake City.[29]

As Voy noted, the increasing commercialisation of modern sports has been associated with massive increases in the financial rewards available to successful athletes. In 1995, Michael Jordan's salary from the Chicago Bulls was $3.9 million but, substantial though this was, it was dwarfed by his earnings from product endorsement, estimated to be in the region of $40 million.[30]

In their history of sports in America since 1945, Roberts and Olsen[31] draw attention to some of the changes in the broader economic and political context within which sport is played. They note that, particularly after 1945, Americans "came to take sports very seriously, and they watched and played for the highest economic, politic, and personal stakes".

The changes described by Roberts and Olsen have not been confined to the United States. In almost all countries, sport is now more competitive and more serious than it used to be. A greater stress is laid upon the importance of winning. And sport is played for higher stakes, whether economic, political, or personal. This is an important part of the context for an understanding of the increasing cooperation between athletes and sports physicians in the search for medal-winning and record-breaking performances; it is, as we have noted, also an important part of the context for understanding the increasing use of drugs within sport.

The sport–medicine axis

It is important to emphasise that sports medicine is a legitimate specialist area of practice and that there is a perfectly proper basis for the increasingly close cooperation between athletes and sports physicians. It is also important to emphasise that there is no evidence to suggest that the great majority of sports physicians behave in anything other than an ethical manner. Notwithstanding this comment, however, it is clear that, at the elite level, the involvement of team doctors in doping is not uncommon and that it has not been confined to the former communist countries of eastern Europe.[7] Among many documented examples of the involvement of team physicians in doping is that concerning the blood doping of the United States cycling team at the 1984 Olympics. Cramer[32] noted: "in the national euphoria after the games, no one thought to pry out any secrets. The US team had won nine medals, dominating the cycling events. 'Great riders...', 'Great coach...', 'Great bikes...', said the press, reporting the daisy chain of back pats. No one thought to add, 'Great doctors...'".

Professional cycling also provides perhaps the clearest example of a "culture of tolerance" in relation to doping; in such situations, the widespread use of drugs is both generally known and tolerated by those involved in the sport. Particularly revealing in this regard was the fact that although the investigation by French police clearly revealed how widespread the practice of doping was in the 1998 Tour de France, no rider failed any drug test carried out by the Tour organisers. Such data raise serious questions about testing procedures and about those responsible for carrying out those procedures.

The Dubin Commission[3] noted: "Many, many more athletes than those actually testing positive have taken advantage of banned substances", and that "positive test results represent only a small proportion of actual drug users". In this regard, it should be noted that several informed observers, including reputable sports journalists (for example Butcher and Nichols, cited in Waddington[7]), senior sports physicians who have held major positions of responsibility (for example, Voy[11]), and elite-level athletes (for example Kimmage,[33] Reiterer[34]) have all argued that senior sports administrators often collude with drug-using athletes to beat the testing system. It may also be the case that, at the elite level, some drug-using athletes are often able to beat the testing system as a result of their access to expert advice from team doctors or other physicians.

As long ago as 1988, the Lancet[35] published an editorial under the title *Sports medicine – is there lack of control?* It suggested that although "evidence of direct involvement of medical practitioners in the procurement and administration of hormones is lacking, their connivance with those who do so is obvious and their participation in blood doping is a matter of record". It concluded that sports medicine should be brought under the umbrella of a recognised body within an accredited programme of professional training. This, it argued, would curb the activities of those few doctors whose interests were more in discovering new ways to enhance an athlete's performance than in looking after their wellbeing.

Two years later, the Dubin Commission of Inquiry in Canada documented the systematic and organised involvement in doping of substantial numbers of sports physicians in many sports and in several countries. The doping scandal surrounding the Tour de France cycle race in 1998 once again provided clear evidence of the systematic and organised involvement of team doctors.[7] Clearly this is a matter of concern not only to the medical profession, but also to all those concerned about doping in sport.

The regulation of doping

Although athletes have for some 2000 years used substances believed to enhance their performance, anti-doping controls within sport were only introduced in the 1960s.[9,36] The first compulsory Olympic drug testing took place at the 1968 Winter Games at Grenoble, and since then anti-doping policies in sport have been based on what might be described as a "law and order" approach, in which emphasis has been placed on the detection and punishment of offenders.

How successful have such policies been? This question is not easy to answer, not least because the objectives of anti-doping policies are rarely clearly defined. However, the following points should be noted in any attempt to evaluate the effectiveness of such policies.

First, Voy[11] has drawn attention to what he calls a "sad paradox" of anti-doping policies. He notes that the severe punishments that often follow the detection of drug use constrain drug-using athletes to place primary importance on the detectability of drugs rather than on their safety; as a consequence, athletes have been pushed towards the use of drugs which may be more dangerous but less detectable.

Secondly, it has been argued[37] that the ban on the use of performance-enhancing drugs makes it difficult for users to obtain medical advice and monitoring in relation to their use of drugs. This consideration may not apply to drug-using elite athletes who work in cooperation with team physicians, but it is certainly the case that at the non-elite level there is an unmet medical need from drug users for qualified, confidential, and non-judgemental medical advice.[38] As stated earlier, the GMC guidance for doctors is:

Doctors who prescribe or collude in the provision of drugs or treatment with the intention of improperly enhancing an individual's performance in sport would be contravening the GMC's guidance, and such actions would usually raise a question of a doctor's continued registration. This does not preclude the provision of any care or treatment where the doctor's intention is to protect or improve the patient's health.[39]

Thirdly, there is no evidence to suggest that the ban on doping has effectively controlled the use of performance-enhancing drugs. Anti-doping policy is discussed in more depth in the next chapter.

Summary

The true extent of doping in elite-level sport is unknown, but evidence suggests that it is much greater than official figures show, and it has increased significantly in the last 50 years. There are a number of reasons that may account for this increase, including the medicalisation of sport, new pressures faced by the athletes, and the increasing competitiveness, commercialisation, and politicisation of sport. Anti-doping policy and controls have not been effective in curbing the activity to date, and so it is imperative that they are critically re-examined.

References

1 Todd T. Anabolic steroids: The gremlins of sport. *J Sport History* 1987;**14**: 87–107.

2 Coni P, Kelland G, Davies D. *AAA Drug abuse enquiry report*. Amateur Athletics Association, 1988.

3 Dubin CL. *Commission of inquiry into the use of drugs and banned practices intended to increase athletic performance*. Ottawa: Canadian Government Publishing Centre, 1990.

4 Australian Parliament. *Drugs in Sport: an interim report of the Senate Standing Committee on Environment, Recreation and the Arts*. Commonwealth of Australia, 1989.

5 Millar AP. Drugs in sport. *J Performance Enhancing Drugs* 1996;**1**: 106–12.

6 Sports Council. *Doping control in the UK: A survey of the experiences and views of elite competitors, 1995*. London: Sports Council, 1996.

7 Waddington I. *Sport, health and drugs*. London and New York: E&FN Spon, 2000.

8 Lenehan P, Bellis M, McVeigh J. A study of anabolic steroid use in the North West of England. *J Performance Enhancing Drugs* 1996;**1**: 57–70.

9 Houlihan B. *Dying to win: Doping in sport and the development of anti-doping policy*. Strasbourg: Council of Europe, 1999.

10 UK Sport. *Doping in sport under the spotlight*. UK Sport latest anti-doping news, 18 June 2001.

11 Voy R. *Drugs, sport and politics*. Champaign, IL: Leisure Press, 1991.

12 British Medical Association. *Sport and exercise medicine: Policy and provision*. London: BMA, 1996.

13 Hoberman J. *Mortal engines*. New York: Free Press, 1992.

14 Brown TC, Benner C. The nonmedical use of drugs. In: Scott WN, Nisonson B, Nicholas JA, eds. *Principles of Sports Medicine*. Baltimore and London: Williams & Wilkins, 1984.

15 Crabbe T. And he's scored: cultures of recreational drug use in football. *J Performance Enhancing Drugs* 1998;**2**: 6–13.

16 Roderick M, Waddington I, Parker G. Playing hurt: Managing injuries in professional football. *Int Rev Sociol Sport* 2000;**35**: 165–80.

17 Waddington I, Roderick M, Parker G. *Managing injuries in professional football: The roles of the club doctor and physiotherapist.* Centre for Research into Sport and Society, University of Leicester, 1999.
18 Donohoe T, Johnson N. *Foul play: Drug abuse in sports.* Oxford: Blackwell Scientific Publications, 1986.
19 Donnelly P. Problems associated with youth involvement in high-performance sport. In: Cahill BR, Pearl AJ, eds. *Intensive Participation in Children's Sports.* Champaign, Illinois: Human Kinetics Publishers, 1993.
20 Sports Coach UK. *Code of conduct for sports coaches.* Leeds: Sports Coach UK, 2001.
21 CASA National Commission on Sports and Substance Abuse. *Winning at any cost: Doping in Olympic sports.* New York: University of Columbia, CASA, 2000.
22 Dunning E, Sheard K. *Barbarians, Gentlemen and Players.* Oxford: Martin Robertson, 1979.
23 Guttmann A. *The Olympics: A history of the modern games.* Urbana and Chicago: University of Illinois Press, 1992.
24 Hill CR. *Olympic Politics.* Manchester and New York: Manchester University Press, 1992.
25 Franke WW, Berendonk B. Hormonal doping and androgenization of athletes: a secret program of the German Democratic Republic government. *Clin Chem* 1997;**43**: 1262–79.
26 On the Line. *Drugs, lies and finishing tape.* BBC2 TV, 24 January 1990.
27 European Group on Ethics in Science and New Technologies. *Opinion on the ethical aspects arising from doping in sport.* Brussels: 1999.
28 Gratton C, Taylor P. *Economics of sport and recreation.* London and New York: E&FN Spon, 2000.
29 International Olympic Committee. Olympic Marketing. *Marketing Matters: The Olympic Marketing Newsletter* 2001;**19**: 3.
30 Armstrong EA. The commodified 23, or, Michael Jordan as text. *Sociol Sport J* 1996;**13**: 325–43.
31 Roberts R, Olsen J. *Winning is the only thing.* Baltimore: Johns Hopkins University Press, 1989.
32 Cramer RB. Olympic cheating: the inside story of illicit doping and the US cycling team. *Rolling Stone* 1985;**441**: 25–26, 30.
33 Kimmage P. *Rough ride: Behind the wheel with a pro cyclist.* London: Yellow Jersey Press, 1998.
34 Reiterer W. *Positive.* Sydney: Pan Macmillan Australia, 2000.
35 Anonymous. Sports medicine – is there lack of control? *Lancet* 1988;**2**: 612.
36 Verroken M. Drug use and abuse in sport. In: Mottram DR, ed., *Drugs in Sport*, 2nd edn. London: E&FN Spon, 1996.
37 Black T. Does the ban on drugs in sport improve societal welfare? *Int Rev Sociol Sport* 1996;**31**: 367–84.
38 Korkia PK, Stimson GV. *Anabolic Steroid Use in Great Britain: an exploratory investigation.* The Centre for Research on Drugs and Health Behaviour. A report for the Department of Health, the Welsh Office and the Chief Scientist Office. Scottish Home and Health Department, 1993.
39 British National Formulary Number 41. London: BMA and RPSGB, 2001.

6: Policy instruments to prevent the use of drugs in sport

Barriers to an effective anti-doping policy

The search for effective responses to social problems is fundamental to public policy. In an ideal world problems would be self-evident, solutions would be based on a detailed understanding of the issues, objectives would be clear and progress toward them measurable, and there would be lasting commitment from policy makers. Yet most problems, such as doping in sport, are often poorly defined and constantly evolving; policy solutions are frequently selected on the basis of a poor understanding of the problem, or because they fulfil some other need, such as that for a quick, cheap, and visible response; objectives are frequently poorly specified and sometimes not specified at all; and evaluation of implementation is rarely budgeted for.

Definition of anti-doping policy

Over the past two decades international anti-doping policies have reflected an attitude that the problem is under control. The consequence of this pattern of policy making is that it has obstructed proper reflection on the nature of the problem and due consideration of the resources needed for the development and implementation of an effective anti-doping policy. The most telling illustration of the complexity at the heart of the issue of doping, is the continuing problem of arriving at an agreed definition of doping in sport (as discussed in Chapter 1). Justice Dubin,[1] Chair of the Canadian Commission of Enquiry into Doping, concluded that a definition of doping was "impossible to achieve", and expressed agreement with Sir Arthur Gold's comment that "The definition lies not in the words but in integrity of character" (quoted in Dubin[1]). Unfortunately, in these increasingly litigious times a precisely worded definition is essential, not only to withstand legal challenge, but also to provide guidance for those tasked with making and implementing anti-doping policy.

Yet agreement on a definition has so far proved elusive, with the IOC and the major international federations producing definitions that variously emphasise danger to health, intent, as well as simply the presence of a banned substance in the body. In a review of the anti-doping rules of 33 international federations, Vrijman[2] found that not only was there little consistency between sports, but that almost all of them were vulnerable to legal challenge. Gay[3] has demonstrated the vulnerability to legal challenge of definitions based on criteria such as "intent" or "use in competition".

In recent years there has been a trend towards "strict liability" definitions, according to which an athlete can be found guilty of a doping infraction "without the sport's governing body proving culpable intent, knowledge or fault; or without the athlete being allowed to prove he or she was faultless".[4] The current IAAF Handbook states that the "offence of doping takes place when ... a prohibited substance is found to be present within an athlete's body tissue or fluids".[5]* The current IOC definition is a little broader, but also includes a strict liability definition: "Doping is i. the use of an expedient (substance or method) which is potentially harmful to athletes' health and/or capable of enhancing their performance, or ii. the presence in the athlete's body of a prohibited substance or evidence of the use thereof or evidence of the use of a prohibited method".[6] Although the IAAF has stuck steadfastly to its strict liability definition, sanctions based on the concept have been rejected by courts in the United States and Switzerland, and by the German track and field legal committee. However, the IAAF has argued strongly that there is no definition of doping which is flawless, and that the strict liability definition is more secure than having to prove intent, harm to the athlete's health, or ergogenic effect.

Identifying the objectives of the policy

If the initial step in policy making – that of defining the problem – continues to prove problematic, it is only one in a series of difficulties facing policy makers. A second concern is to agree the objectives of the anti-doping policy. How much of the spectrum that runs from Olympic sports through to unorganised, individual non-sports-oriented activities such as vanity bodybuilding should the anti-doping

---

* Two other clauses in the IAAF Handbook refer to doping methods and the admission of drug use.

campaign embrace? Should all drugs and sports be treated as deserving equal attention, or should the use of β blockers in archery be deemed to be less serious than the use of human growth hormone in swimming? Finally, what are realistic goals for an anti-doping policy – a reduction in the experimentation with new drugs, a reduction in the quantity of illegal drugs used, a reduction in drug abuse in particular sports or at particular events, or drug-free sport?

Budget setting

A third difficulty follows from the last question and concerns the extent of public resources that can be justified in pursuit of anti-doping policy goals. In some countries the budget for supporting the anti-doping effort is almost as large as that devoted to the promotion of mass participation, and is growing more rapidly: the escalating opportunity cost of supporting the anti-doping campaign is likely to be challenged with increasing vigour in the coming years. The estimated cost of developing and validating the test for erythropoietin (EPO) was thought to be in the region of £3m. However, just as a reliable test for EPO has been developed, rumours are circulating of the use by athletes of a new drug, Hemopure, with claims that it has a similar effect to EPO but, as a polymerised haemoglobin, contains no red blood cells and will require the development of a new test. Although Hemopure is scientifically detectable, there are as yet no internationally approved tests for sport.

Legal challenges

Fourth, there is the increasing threat of legal challenge to the decisions of anti-doping authorities. In many sports elite athletes are richer than their domestic governing body, and although legal action might be expensive for the athlete, it might be crippling for the governing body. The court action by Diane Modahl contributed to the bankruptcy of the British Athletic Federation (BAF), and the successor to the BAF, UK Athletics, has been accused by the IAAF of failing to penalise drug users because of the fear of legal challenge. Few domestic governing bodies possess a sufficiently healthy financial base to afford a prolonged court case even if successful, and fewer could afford the cost of defeat in the courts. Although some have suggested that the government should assume the financial risk of legal action, it has understandably been reluctant to do so.

Scientific controversies

A fifth problem arises from the number of scientific controversies that persist, which include the use of blood testing and the difficulty in distinguishing exogenous from endogenous hormone. Blood sampling has already been used on a limited basis in skiing, track and field, and cycling, and was cleared for use at the 2000 Sydney Olympics in the detection of EPO, albeit in conjunction with traditional urine testing. It is also currently under investigation as a test for human growth hormone. Despite the growing evidence of the efficacy of blood sampling and the legitimacy given to it by its adoption at Sydney, there remain a number of unresolved ethical and legal issues concerning its use.

Among the issues to be considered are the following. Blood sampling is new to many athletes; it is invasive and may therefore cause anxiety and pain; unlike urine, blood is not a waste product; on-site processing of blood samples may be required; blood sampling involves a slight risk of infection to the donor and to the sampling officer and other staff; and venepuncture requires trained staff. To date, there has been no challenge to blood sampling in the UK courts, but a challenge might be possible on the grounds that it may breach the European Convention on Human Rights (those rights under Articles* 3, 8, 9 and 10) and the Convention on Human Rights and Biomedicine (with regard to Articles** 5 and 10). Any medical practitioners who do carry out sampling should be aware of the possibility, albeit remote, of a challenge on human rights grounds. In some countries (Austria, for example) blood sampling for non-medical purposes is illegal. In others, the analysis of a blood sample comes under public health legislation, which requires the notification of any infectious diseases discovered during analysis, and which imposes controls on the movement of blood across national boundaries. However, as a number of sports administrators have pointed out, regular blood sampling is part of the testing regimen to assess the effectiveness of training in many, if not most, elite athletes, and is therefore far from being a novelty.

---

* Article 3: The right to freedom from torture and inhuman or degrading treatment or punishment.
Article 8: The right to respect for private and family life, home, and correspondence.
Article 9: The right to freedom of thought, conscience, and religion.
Article 10: The right to freedom of expression.
** Article 5: General rule on the issue of consent.
Article 10: Private life and the right to information.

The problems of distinguishing between exogenous and endogenous hormone is best illustrated by the current confusion surrounding nandrolone, which has gained public attention owing to the sharp rise in the number of positive tests for the drug, up from four in 1998 to 17 in 1999. In the UK a number of high-profile athletes have tested positive for nandrolone. This sharp rise prompted UK Sport to convene a panel to review current procedures for the analysis of the drug. The study, led by Professor Vivian James, confirmed the reliability of current testing and analytical procedures. However, the Nandrolone Review Committee did identify the need for "clarification by the IOC of the 'upper limit of normal' of nandrolone detection [of 2 nanograms per millilitre of urine for males and 5 for females] and the basis for determining laboratory reporting levels".[7] The Committee is continuing to look at the issue.

It is suggested that the upper limits set for a number of other drugs are also based on weak scientific evidence and are consequently vulnerable to legal challenge.

The extent of disagreement over the threshold for declaring a positive result is illustrated by a dispute between FIFA and the IOC. FIFA reported that a study it had commissioned of 148 Swiss soccer players showed that players could exceed the IOC threshold for nandrolone when under stress. However, these findings were rejected by Professor Christine Ayotte, head of the IOC-accredited laboratory in Montreal, who argued that the conclusions drawn by FIFA not only exceeded the scope of the study, but also contradicted the findings of more extensive studies carried out at the Nagano Winter Olympics and the 1999 PanAm Games.

Reasons for athlete non-compliance

The number and complexity of problems facing anti-doping policy makers are compounded by the variety of causes of non-compliance. Table 6.1 demonstrates that the success of each policy instrument will depend on the cause of non-compliance. The table also draws attention to the range of policies available ranging from inducements at one end to sanctions at the other.

Table 6.1 takes as its focus the causes of non-compliance among adult athletes. In the UK context, and indeed internationally since the collapse of communism in central Europe, few athletes could claim that they were prevented from complying with anti-doping regulations, despite the fact that some argue that they are under considerable

Table 6.1 Causes of non-compliance with anti-doping rules and the likely effectiveness of policy instruments.

Cause of non-compliance by athlete	Policy instruments			
	Rewards (for example money and public honours)	Information/education (for example on banned substances and practices, and also on the health effects of sustained use)	Erection of barriers (for example control of the supply of drugs)	Deterrents (for example extensive testing, fines, and periods of suspension from competition)
Ignorance or incompetence	Negligible	Substantial potential effect	Moderate	Negligible
Inability to comply (lack of free will)	Negligible	Negligible	Moderate	Negligible
Conscious decision not to comply	Moderate	Moderate	Moderate	Moderate to substantial

pressure from their entourage and from their peers to take drugs. In cases where athletes lack the freedom to make choices, policies that are directed at individual athletes are unlikely to be successful. Ignorance or incompetence are more plausible causes of non-compliance, given the complexity of the IOC list of banned substances and practices, the fact that it changed annually until 2000 and subsequently will change biannually, and the varying levels of sophistication awareness among athletes. It is in this area that the provision of information and the establishment of education programmes would be most effective. Finally, where anti-doping agencies are faced by athletes who decide not to comply – which is likely to be the largest group of non-compliers in the UK – then a combination of policies might be employed, designed to restrict supply, deter use through the extent and effectiveness of the testing programme, and provide information on the effects of long-term use of drugs.

Even taking one target group produces a fairly complex pattern of possible policies. The complexity is compounded when the adult group is disaggregated by sport or gender, for example, and when additional target groups are considered, such as young athletes (minors), coaches and other members of the athlete's entourage, and national governing bodies. It would be possible to rework Table 6.1 for each of these groups, thereby producing a series of bespoke policy responses. For example, although few adult athletes could claim to be *unable* to comply, this is a much more plausible cause of non-compliance among minors. The importance of young people as a target group for policy is evident from a recent Sport England survey of 12 sports, which showed that the average age at which athletes entered sport at the performance level was 11 years 6 months, and that on average athletes in six sports (women's and men's judo, swimming, netball, women's hockey, and sailing) moved to elite-level competition before the age of 18.

The global nature of sport

A further complication arises from the global nature of the problem, reflected in the international nature of sports competition and the geographical mobility of athletes. Many of the UK's elite athletes will undertake most of their competition outside the UK, and outside the immediate jurisdiction of their domestic governing body. In addition, many athletes will train, for part of the year at least, abroad. Consequently, any attempt at strengthening and refining domestic anti-doping policy needs to be complemented by an equal effort to develop and enhance policy at the international level.

Are current policies focused on the right people?

Among other problems with current policy is one that more directly affects the medical profession. This relates to the fact that since the introduction of anti-doping policies in the 1960s, such policies have focused almost exclusively on the individual drug-using athlete and, as the Dubin Commission[1] noted, "no effort was made to ascertain if others were involved. The obvious people – coaches, doctors, trainers – were simply ignored". This policy is unrealistic. There is now an abundance of evidence to indicate that, at least at the elite level, the drug-using athlete is normally part of a network of relationships with others. This may include team members, coaches, doctors, masseurs, trainers, managers, or promoters, who are involved in supplying or administering doping substances, or in concealing their use. The highly individualistic perspective that has been underlying anti-doping policy is not only based on a misunderstanding of the social relations involved in the doping process, but it also focuses exclusively on the wrongdoing of one individual while ignoring the wrongdoing of others who are heavily implicated. This is a matter which needs to be addressed by the IOC and governing bodies within sport.

However, there are examples of organisations outside those responsible for establishing anti-doping policies that have made a stand against doping. As discussed earlier, British doctors risk being struck off the medical register by the General Medical Council if they are found to be involved in doping. Coaches who are members of Sports Coach UK, the national coaching foundation, must abide by a code of conduct which stipulates that coaches must educate athletes on issues relating to the use of performance-enhancing drugs in sports and cooperate fully with UK Sport and national governing body (NGB) policies. It aims to support NGBs in implementing the code by assisting in developing appropriate policies and procedures for dealing with allegations and complaints based on coaching practice.

Choosing policy instruments

The review of evidence outlined in Chapter 5 suggests that doping is widespread in many sports, and that in some sports it is very widespread. If it can be assumed that a central objective of anti-doping policies is to control the use of performance-enhancing drugs by athletes, then it would seem reasonable to conclude that current anti-doping policy has not worked well. This is not to suggest that anti-doping controls to date should be dismantled and that athletes should be allowed to take any substances without regulation; apart from health-related objections to such a policy, an extremely liberal policy of this kind is simply not politically realistic. However, there are a number of other policy options that might be explored.

Deterrence

The early years of anti-doping policy were characterised by the belief among sports administrators and many governments that doping was the activity of a very small minority, that it was a more serious problem in other sports or other countries, and that in-competition testing was an effective deterrent. This perception of the problem created a mould for future policy which identified testing and sanctions as the defining elements of policy. To some extent this approach also reflected the existing attitude towards recreational drug use, where the most common policy is one of suppression of demand through deterrent punishments. It is only recently that policy makers have acknowledged the heterogeneity of the problem and have begun to identify a broader range of policy instruments from which to construct a more tailored response. Few policies are based exclusively on one of the four types of policy instruments identified in Table 6.1, and anti-doping policy is unusual in relying so heavily on deterrence. Attempts to reduce the excessive consumption of alcohol, for example, combine education programmes, the erection of barriers (such as the licensing of sales outlets), and deterrents (for example high excise duties).

Unfortunately, despite the emphasis given to deterrence over the last 30 years, the policy instrument is far from coherent or effective. The harmonisation of sanctions has been a priority of policy makers for some time and is high on the agenda of the World Anti-Doping Agency (WADA). The 1999 IOC Anti-Doping Code attempted to achieve a greater degree of uniformity between Olympic sports. The Code divided drugs into two categories, one that included less serious drugs, such as ephedrine, caffeine, and phenylpropanolamine, whose use incurred a penalty ranging from a warning to suspension from competition for six months, and one that included the more serious drugs, such as steroids, where the penalty ranged from a ban on participation in one or several competitions to suspension for two years. For a second offence involving a drug from either category the penalty ranged from a four-year ban to a life ban.

A particular difficulty in achieving the level of harmonisation sought by the IOC is the preference for treating all (Olympic) sports in the same way. Some international federations – those for cycling and athletics – adapted the IOC list of banned substances and practices to suit the peculiarities of their sport, but most federations simply adopted the IOC list without amendment, an action which was less an indication of satisfaction with the list than a reflection of a lack of resources to make an independent judgement, or possibly simply apathy. However, as the debate on harmonisation of sanctions intensified a number of federations began to express a reluctance to accept the IOC preference for a minimum sanction of two years for a serious doping offence. Football and tennis have been among the more reluctant federations, with FIFA being the most vociferous in its refusal to adhere to the two-year standard. As a result the 1999 IOC Code contains the following clause relating to offences involving a more serious drug offence: "...the penalties for a first offence are as follows: ... suspension from any competition for a minimum period of two years. However, based on specific, exceptional circumstances to be evaluated in the first instance by the competent IF [International Federation] bodies, there may be a provision for a possible modification of the two-year sanction".[6]

There is a clear danger that agreement on a common minimum period of suspension will only be achieved by seeking out the lowest common denominator which, if the aim is to include all the major sports, might be set at a very low level indeed. It might be possible to place a more positive gloss on the current impasse on sanctions by arguing that the aim of the IOC should not be to establish a range of penalties that are treated as a norm, but rather to establish a minimum tariff and then encourage sports federations to create a set of bespoke penalties that suit the particular characteristics of their sport. For example, a two-year suspension from competition represents a greater proportion of the elite career of a female gymnast than that of a male rower. A two-year suspension is also much more significant to an athlete at the peak of his or her career than to one just breaking through to international level. However, such a view assumes too great a degree of enthusiasm to tackle doping among international federations.

International federations that might be inclined to set a penalty above the IOC minimum of two years for serious offences have not been encouraged by the experience of the IAAF, whose decision to suspend the runner Katrin Krabbe for three years was overturned by the Munich Regional Appeal Court, which claimed that "more than two years contravene ... the constitutional principle of proportionality".[8,9] A further difficulty undermining sanctions as an effective policy instrument is the growing reluctance among domestic governing bodies to impose sanctions. In the UK there has been a series of positive drug tests in athletics where the governing body, UK Athletics, has concluded that a doping infraction has not taken place, only for the decision to be overturned by the IAAF.

The substantial weaknesses that remain in the development of sanctions as a policy instrument should not detract from the progress that has been made in recent years in achieving a greater degree of harmonisation, nor from the momentum that has been added to the search for harmonisation, by the establishment of WADA. Nevertheless, it is clear that to construct a policy response to doping around sanctions alone would be unwise, even if the remaining problems could be resolved. Although the issue of sanctions continues to dominate the agenda, there have been attempts to establish a more broadly based policy which utilises other instruments, such as education.

Education

The designers of education programmes need to address a series of issues if they are to feel confident that the programmes will be effective:

1. Select the appropriate target groups, which might include governing bodies, various categories of athletes (such as junior, senior, veteran, male, female), coaches, parents, team/squad doctors, sponsors, and so forth.
2. Determine the attitudes of the various groups towards doping.
3. Understand what these various groups know about doping and doping control procedures.
4. Identify their information sources and their reliability.
5. Determine the medium (text or video, for example) and the "voice" (for example doctors, scientists, or top athletes) that would be the most successful.
6. Agree the message, or combination of messages, likely to be the most effective – for example damage to health, appeal to fair play, threat of suspension, loss of income, poor example set to the young.

Although there have been useful surveys of athletes, young people, coaches, and doctors, there is still remarkably little research into these issues and questions. Many surveys are of athletes and are intended to determine the extent of doping at elite level which, though important, is only of limited value in guiding policy. Among the more interesting of these surveys is that by the Australian Sports Drug Agency[10] undertaken in 1994, which collected data on the level of awareness of the work of the Agency, especially its educational programme, among athletes. It was found, inter alia, that awareness of ASDA was high and that elite athletes perceived the general effectiveness of international testing as low.

In Britain, the Sports Council published a survey in 1995 which covered similar ground to that of ASDA and which provided some valuable data on where elite athletes obtained their information on doping. Interestingly, 72% of elite athletes, when ill, had received advice on allowable medicines when they approached their national governing body doctor, but only 54% had received similar advice from their general practitioner.[11] A more recent survey by The Netherlands Centre for Doping (NeCeDo)[12] of over 1300 elite Dutch athletes was carried out in 1999. The findings disclosed a high level of ignorance of doping control procedures, particularly among young athletes; a high level of support for tougher penalties for doping infractions; a high degree of ignorance and uncertainty about the use of dietary supplements; and a lack of knowledge about the role of the Dutch anti-doping agency, NeCeDo.

The Canadian Centre for Drug-Free Sport undertook a national survey of students aged between 11 and 18 which revealed that different approaches were required for younger and older athletes, that knowledge of the health risks of steroid use was a weak deterrent, and that coaches and older athletes are particularly influential in shaping the attitudes of the young athlete.[13]

There are also some surveys of the attitudes and behaviour of doctors. A 1997 survey of 7000 Dutch GPs by NeCeDo found that 280 either had prescribed or were prepared to prescribe banned drugs to their patients.[14] This supports an earlier French study by Laure,[15] in which it was reported that 61% of amateur athletes who admitted using drugs obtained them from their GP, some reportedly with the full knowledge of the doctor.

The Australian Sports Drug Agency (ASDA)[16] in 1996 undertook a survey of coaches which sought to gather information about their understanding of doping issues, their involvement in anti-doping efforts, and their knowledge of the work of ASDA. The survey concluded that although coaches were supportive of the work of ASDA, they lacked specific knowledge of its role: over 40% either never or rarely talked about doping issues with their athletes; and although 93% and 98% respectively correctly identified stimulants and anabolic steroids as banned substances, only 52% correctly identified the status of β agonists and 60% the status of local anaesthetics.

One attempt to develop an educational resource for use in combating doping was prepared jointly by the Council of Europe and the European Union. *The Clean Sport Guide*[17] is designed to support the development of anti-doping educational programmes in member countries. The first section of the *Guide* provides much useful advice on the steps to be taken in developing an educational programme and also provides a list of examples of good practice. The *Guide* is a rich resource and one that could ideally be used by national anti-doping agencies in conjunction with individual governing bodies to develop targeted policy. One theme that runs through the *Guide* is the need for educational campaigns to be based on a secure understanding of the problem.

There are also a number of examples of publicity campaigns designed to promote an anti-doping ethos, such as the "True

Champions" campaign launched in 2000 by ASDA. Using a variety of media, ASDA sums up its message to the athlete as being "to achieve your best through hard work and dedication without using banned drugs, to work within your sport to preserve its value; and to honour the faith your family and friends place in you by doing what's right".[18] ASDA has also developed a series of bespoke education programmes for individual sports. Canada has for some time promoted a "Spirit of Sport" campaign which has organised events and publicity relating to aspects of ethical sport, including drug-free sport.

Finally, there is also a need, recognised by the UK Sport Anti-Doping Directorate (ADD), for the development of education programmes and resources for drug-abusing athletes who are serving a period of suspension. Such a programme should seek to ensure, as far as is possible, that they return to their sport with a revised set of personal values, in much the same way that education is sometimes part of the rehabilitation process for serious social drug abusers and alcoholics.

In summary, our knowledge of why people take drugs in sport is based more on assertion and intuition than research. We also know little about how motives for drug use vary between sports, genders, ages, and status. There is also little research into which, if any, educational initiatives, such as those based on *The Clean Sport Guide*, have been successful. Some parallels can be drawn with educational campaigns regarding the use of recreational drugs, tobacco, and alcohol, but there are few data related specifically to the unique aspects of the problem of doping in sport.

Barriers

The third general policy instrument mentioned in Table 6.1 is the erection of barriers to undesirable behaviour. In the case of doping, the most obvious example of this strategy would be an attempt to control the supply of banned substances. However, many banned substances are available over the counter in pharmacies, and others, such as anabolic steroids, despite being subject to legal control, are available in such variety and from so many manufacturers and suppliers that monitoring and control of supply is not practicable. There are, though, a number of drugs, such as human growth hormone and Hemopure (a polymerised haemoglobin), where a tighter control over supply may be feasible. These are drugs where therapeutic use and the number of manufacturers are both limited. It is perfectly feasible for manufacturers to keep a closer check on the distribution of their products, or to include in the drug a marker that would ease detection in the laboratory analysis of urine samples. Whether the pharmaceutical companies would cooperate would depend on the extent to which they perceived the leakage of their products from orthodox use to illegal use in sport as a threat to their integrity, or as a welcome additional source of profit. It would also make access to drugs more difficult if there was an effective process in the UK for analysing the number of prescriptions written for steroids, for example, and for tracing them back to individual GPs. Although there is such a system for the analysis of prescriptions on the NHS (prescribing analysis and cost, or PACT), there is no such system for private prescriptions.

Incentives and rewards

The final major policy instrument mentioned in Table 6.1 is the use of incentives and rewards. Through the annual presentation of Canadian Sports Awards, Canada rewards its athletes on the basis of their behaviour as well as their sporting achievements. In addition to the presentation of awards, ASDA also encourages athletes to carry a drug test passport. ASDA launched the "True Champion Passport" in summer 2000, a voluntary scheme that enables athletes to demonstrate their commitment to drug-free sport. Passports are updated regularly with the testing history of the athlete. If the scheme is successful, athletes will be required to possess a validated passport with an adequate history to be able to compete or to return to competition after a period of suspension for a doping infraction. The UK Anti-Doping Directorate (ADD) supports a drug passport scheme in principle, and currently encourages athletes to fill in their test details in the space provided at the back of the "Competitors and Officials Guide to Drugs in Sport" (Verroken M, personal communication 2001).

Harm reduction policy

As Coomber[19] has noted, many of the public health issues involved in the use of drugs in sport are not dissimilar to those involved in the use of drugs in a non-sporting context. Thus athletes "may be using unsafe ways of administering their drugs, using unsafe drugs in unsafe ways, and may even be unintentional transmission routes into the non-sporting world of sexually transmitted diseases such as HIV".[19] Outside the sporting context, public health authorities in many countries have sought to deal with problems of this kind by the development of "harm reduction" policies. Coomber describes the development of these policies in Britain as follows:

With the advent of HIV/AIDS in the non-sporting world, drug policy concerned itself with reducing the spread of HIV to the general population. This meant accessing one of the high-risk groups likely to spread the virus-injecting drug users – who had contracted high levels of infection due to needle-sharing practices. Access to this group, and introducing them to practices likely to reduce the spread of the virus took priority over compelling these people to stop using drugs. Without access to non-judgemental help and real benefits (such as clean needles, and in some circumstances even access to drugs of choice), these users, who were not interested in stopping using drugs, would not have been accessed. A major policy decision was made that HIV represented a bigger threat to Public Health than drug use".[19]

Harm reduction includes a variety of strategies, with needle exchange schemes a central aspect of such policies. Rather than attempting to eliminate drug use – an unrealistic target – the goal is to reduce harm. Harm reduction policies are already well established in a number of countries, including The Netherlands, Switzerland, and Britain,[20] and some aspects of US policy, for example the methadone maintenance programmes for heroin addicts, might also be considered as a move away from traditional punitive policies.

However, within the sporting world anti-drugs policy has been almost exclusively of the punitive, "law and order" kind, and little thought has been given to the development of harm reduction policies. Coomber suggests that one reason for this is that those responsible for making and implementing anti-doping policy in sport "do not, in general, work within the same parameters as those policy makers outside sport. Drug policy in sport is seen as an issue that concerns sport and sporting authorities, and it has essentially isolated itself from considerations of how drug policy in sport relates to the world outside of it". He suggests that there are "many lessons to be learned about drugs, drug users and methods of control from the non-sporting world",[19] particularly in relation to harm reduction policies.

What, then, would a harm reduction policy in sport look like, and what might be the advantages of such a policy? This question is not an entirely hypothetical one, for there have been some small but important movements in sport towards harm reduction policies.

One such harm reduction scheme worthy of examination is that in operation in County Durham. In January 1994, the County Durham

Health Authority began funding a mobile needle exchange scheme (also discussed in Chapter 4) which was targeted at injecting drug users and which was designed in the first instance as part of a harm reduction policy in relation to the transmission of HIV infection. To the surprise of the organisers of the needle exchange scheme, it quickly became clear that a majority of those using it were bodybuilders who were using anabolic steroids. Some users of anabolic steroids had been attracted to the scheme because they had been unable to get medical help and advice from their regular physicians, some of whom had responded to requests for help in a hostile and heavily judgemental fashion and had refused to offer any advice until the bodybuilders stopped using steroids. With this evidence of unmet medical need in the area, in early 1995 County Durham Health Authority established a "drugs and sport clinic and users support clinic" (DISCUS).

The clinic has approximately 450 clients, most of whom are bodybuilders (Dawson R, personal communication 2001). It provides a confidential and non-judgemental service to users of anabolic steroids and other performance-enhancing drugs, and the policy goals of the clinic centre around harm reduction rather than cessation of drug use. New clients are given an initial assessment in relation to their pattern of drug use and sexual health (the latter mainly in respect of HIV transmission), followed by a physical examination which includes blood sample analysis for a red blood cell count and a lipid profile. In addition, clients are monitored for liver function. Clients are encouraged to ensure that the intervals between cycles of drug use are such as to minimise the health risks, and are also given advice, for example in relation to diet, which may help them to achieve their desired body shape with lower doses of drugs, or perhaps by using less dangerous drugs. A confidential counselling service is also provided for anabolic steroid users who experience side effects such as sexual dysfunction or aggression.[21] A not dissimilar scheme is run by an agency in the Wirral, Merseyside, which also offers information and support, including monitoring of blood pressure, plasma cholesterol, and liver function, and HIV screening, for users of anabolic steroids. Other schemes are in operation in Nottingham and Cardiff, and an increasing number of agencies have workers in the field targeting anabolic steroid users.[22]

What lessons can be learned from such schemes? Should sporting and/or public medical authorities consider the more widespread funding of such schemes as part of a harm reduction policy? What might be some of the consequences of a reorientation on the part of sporting bodies towards harm reduction policies? And what might be some of the objections to such a shift in policy?

At the outset it should be acknowledged that a reorientation of policy along these lines would not be unproblematic. However, if we are honest we should also recognise that the issue of drug use and control is, as Goode[20] has pointed out, one where there may be no ideal solution, and that it may well be that we are forced to accept "the least bad of an array of very bad options".

Possible objections to harm reduction policies

One possible objection to harm reduction policies is that such policies, it might be argued, imply condoning the use of drugs. In response to possible objections of this kind, it might be noted that such arguments were also voiced when harm reduction policies, such as needle exchange schemes, were initially developed in relation to drug control policies more generally. Although such arguments are still occasionally heard, the case for needle exchange schemes has now generally been accepted in Britain, and such schemes have been funded by governments – both Conservative and Labour – which no one could legitimately accuse of having adopted a "soft" or permissive policy in relation to drug use in general. Thus the shift towards harm reduction policies is not incompatible with, and does not imply the dismantling of, more conventional forms of drug control.

Possible benefits of harm reduction policies

What health benefits might be associated with harm reduction policies? One obvious benefit associated with "sport and drugs" clinics of the kind outlined above is that they provide what is clearly a much needed service to those using performance-enhancing drugs, whether in sport or other sport-related activities, not least in the fact that they provide qualified, confidential, and non-judgemental medical advice which otherwise might be difficult to obtain. Although many drug-using athletes at the elite level undoubtedly receive qualified medical advice and monitoring, it may be the case that, even at the elite level, there are some who do not receive such support. Moreover, it is clear that below this level there is a considerable unmet demand for medical support. A study carried out in British gymnasiums indicated that users of anabolic steroids generally felt that most medical practitioners had little knowledge of their use, and were unable to provide unbiased information on different drugs and their effects on health. The researchers found that "the majority of AS [anabolic steroid] users would welcome medical involvement but are unable to get the supervision they would like".[22]

Anti-doping policy in the UK

Doping in sport has been a matter of public policy since the mid-1960s in the UK and is currently the responsibility of the Anti-Doping Directorate (ADD) of UK Sport. The UK has long been at the forefront of attempts to tackle doping in sport, and ranks among the leading nations in terms of its current contribution to policy development and implementation, alongside Canada, Australia, France, Norway, and Sweden.

ADD in the UK

The precise role of ADD has been shaped substantially by the increasing internationalisation of the issue and the fact that the major UK national governing bodies (NGBs) of sport have rarely been capable of operating effectively within a global or European policy context. As a result the government, through ADD, has taken the initiative in shaping the increasingly important organisational infrastructure for policy making at the international level.

The current division of labour between the ADD and the NGBs is such that the former provides finance for the bulk of testing and research. The ADD has also taken the initiative in establishing links with doping control agencies in other countries, with a view to strengthening the degree of harmonisation of procedures in relation to testing. The roles of the NGBs are to consult with the ADD concerning the testing programme for their sport (for example the number of tests, and the balance between in-competition and out-of-competition tests) and, most importantly, to determine the consequences of a positive test result for the athlete. The ADD thus fulfils an important but delicate role, at times leading and at other times cajoling the NGBs to take their responsibility for sports ethics seriously.

The changing role and pattern of activity of ADD reflect the rapid changes in the context of anti-doping policy making. Until the late 1980s the prevailing assumption was that the problem of doping could be tackled within a series of relatively discrete areas defined by the boundaries of particular sports, competitions, or countries. The internationalisation of the problem of doping has strained the resources of both governments and sports bodies and has necessitated a substantial readjustment in policy orientation. At the time of writing this report (November 2001), the BMA is aware that UK Sport is planning to launch a revised Statement of Anti-Doping Policy in early 2002. The objective of this draft policy is "to ensure that all governing bodies of sport in the UK have consistent anti-doping policies and regulations to protect the rights of athletes to compete drug free".[23]

ADD in the international arena

The UK was among the first countries to begin to explore an international solution to the problem of doping, helping to form the "Memorandum of Understanding Group", which was later retitled the "International Anti-doping Agreement" (IADA) and which aimed to facilitate the harmonisation of domestic anti-doping procedures and, more importantly, to act as a lobby within the international sports community. ADD is also a strong supporter of the policy efforts of the Council of Europe and is an active member of the "Anti-Doping Convention Monitoring Group". The UK, through ADD, was at the heart of the debates surrounding the formation of the World Anti-Doping Agency (WADA), and has been influential in helping to shape the emerging interest in doping within the European Union. In summary, ADD provides the UK with an influential voice in increasingly crucial international policy-making forums, and provides the UK with a substantial degree of moral authority on matters associated with doping.

UK weaknesses

The UK's and, by implication, ADD's contribution to policy making has been weak, however, in relation to the contribution of its domestic governing bodies (NGBs). UK Athletics in particular has been accused by its parent federation (IAAF) of not taking a sufficiently robust approach to doping infractions. Particularly in relation to cases involving nandrolone, UK Athletics has regularly decided not to treat the positive result as a doping infraction, only for the IAAF to reverse the decision and suspend the athlete. The apparent soft-pedalling by domestic governing bodies is, in large part, due to a fear of litigation, which would be costly even if the decision by the NGB were supported by the court.

With this problem in mind, the government has supported the establishment by the major sports governing bodies in September 1999 of the "Sports Disputes Resolution Panel", an independent not-for-profit company, in an attempt to provide a low-cost alternative to the courts. The Panel is funded by UK Sport for four years, covering the core administrative costs. However, it is evident that the Panel is not what sport needs – that is, a low-cost, convenient, and speedy resolution process – as parties to the dispute will have to pay for a hearing and are likely to feel obliged to employ legal representation. The draft revised Statement of Anti-Doping Policy proposes the appointment of an Independent Scrutiny Committee to oversee the results management process by UK Sport and the NGBs. This aims to ensure that the review process is fair and accurate, and that international concerns about disciplinary actions not being taken by UK governing bodies are addressed.

A second area of weakness with the policy has been the emphasis on deterrence and the interdiction of supply, and the underinvestment in alternative (or at least complementary) policy instruments such as education aimed at culture change and rewards. At this stage of policy making it would be timely to balance existing policy with a greater emphasis on reducing demand. It is in this area that research designed to identify the most effective ways of reducing demand is largely missing in the UK, particularly compared to Canada and Australia. However, there is a clear move within ADD to reorient policy away from its current focus on deterrence and the drug-abusing athletes, and towards a greater concern to protect the rights of drug-free athletes. The 2000 Statement of Anti-Doping Policy moved tentatively in that direction with its stated intention "to protect the right of athletes to participate in drug-free sport",[24] and the draft revised Statement has the same objective, as quoted above. To that end, NGBs will be required, as a condition of their grant, to ensure the effective implementation of the programme derived from the Statement. In fact, under the revised Statement (2002), without an anti-doping policy approved by UK Sport, an NGB will not be recognised by the Sports Councils and hence will not be considered for Lottery or Exchequer funding. The Statement is, above all, an attempt to increase the degree of commitment from NGBs to a professional and rigorous anti-doping programme, and to ensure a greater degree of harmonisation of procedures for dealing with alleged doping infractions. It is difficult to be accepted as a serious participant in international anti-doping policy making unless there is clear evidence of a rigorous policy at home.

A related reorientation of policy that the ADD is seeking to achieve, is to balance sanctions with a policy of rehabilitation for the offending athlete. At present, athletes who receive a suspension are left largely unsupervised during their period outside the sport. NGBs are encouraged to generate a close working relationship with the UK Sports Institute and Athlete Career and Education Programme (ACE) advisors to offer counselling and rehabilitation opportunities.[23,25] It would strengthen the effectiveness of the sanction and its likelihood of altering behaviour if governing bodies were *required* to provide rehabilitation and support for athletes during the period of their suspension. Both the current and draft Statements state only that governing bodies should publish conditions for eligibility for reinstatement, including *whether* an athlete is required to participate in a programme of rehabilitation and education. A programme of rehabilitation could be linked to the idea of an athlete's passport, in which the tests undertaken during rehabilitation and the programme of counselling and so forth would be logged and presented as evidence of fitness for readmission to the sport. UK Sport could work together with the Health Development Agency to establish an effective rehabilitation programme, to which NGBs would then be required to send their athletes in the event that they fail a drugs test, and as part of the reinstatement procedure.

The maintenance of the ADD's position at the forefront of policy innovation, at both domestic and international levels, depends on continued support from other key bodies within UK sport. As stated earlier, at the time of writing (November 2001) we are aware that the ADD will be launching a revised Statement of Anti-Doping Policy early in 2002, with the backing of the government. Prior to this time, it would have been accurate to question the degree of the government's enthusiasm. Although financial support has increased over the last 10 years it has not enabled the ADD to increase significantly the number of tests it funds since 1990, and has certainly not matched the increase in testing in countries such as France. It is also noteworthy that the National Lottery has been used extensively to support the preparation of the UK's elite athletes for competition, but no Lottery funds have been forthcoming for drug testing. Certainly, until the preparation of the revised anti-doping statement, it has not appeared that drug-free sport was central to the government's high-performance sports strategy.

This said, there has been little discussion of the legislative and financial arrangements that will need to be in place for the forthcoming Commonwealth Games. It should be remembered that Australia doubled its expenditure on doping control for the 2000 Olympics. Furthermore, the 2000 nandrolone report and the rise in the number of cases of positive tests for steroids have not prompted any significant expressions of governmental concern to date.

Summary

The overriding impression of anti-doping efforts in the UK has been that government enthusiasm has been intermittent and that many organisations have a conflict of interest. The major governing bodies are in the position of seeking to maximise international success while at the same time rigorously enforcing an anti-doping policy which is certainly perceived by some as a major threat to the achievement of that success. It is certainly questionable whether governing bodies can be both gamekeeper and poacher with equal enthusiasm.

Furthermore, the position of the ADD has not been beyond challenge. Although the Directorate continues to be one of the six or so leading anti-doping agencies in the world, some have asked whether its location within UK Sport is appropriate, as UK Sport is also responsible for the elite development strategy and the attraction of major sports events to the country. It may be argued that this mix of responsibilities will create a tension within the organisation, if not a direct conflict of interest. This has led to the argument that if the government is serious about tackling the issue of doping in sport, it would seem logical to vest responsibility in an independent agency with strong legislative protection: the government must be seen to be in the forefront of setting standards in sport.

However, it would seem that rather than establishing a new agency, the plan is in fact to strengthen UK Sport from within. The revised anti-doping policy statement to be launched early in 2002 appears to have greater commitment from the government, particularly in terms of emphasising UK Sport's accountability to the public. The establishment of an Independent Scrutiny Committee seems to point to a move towards a process built on transparency. The proposed policy of withdrawing the recognition of Sports Councils, and hence even the consideration of Lottery and Exchequer funding, from NGBs that do not have an anti-doping policy, indicates a strengthening of the UK's commitment to the Anti-Doping Convention of the Council of Europe,[26] and to the fight against doping in sport overall. After so many years of variable government commitment to the anti-doping policy, however, it will be interesting to monitor whether this proposed shift in policy emphasis leads to a reduction in the use of drugs in sport, and whether this can be maintained.

References

1 Dubin CL. *Commission of inquiry into the use of drugs and banned practices intended to increase athletic performance.* Ottawa: Canadian Government Publishing Centre, 1990.

2 Vrijman EN. *Harmonisation, can it ever really be achieved?* Strasbourg: Council of Europe, 1995.

3 Gay M. *Constitutional aspects of testing for prohibited substances.* London: Unpublished paper, not dated.

4 Wise AN. Strict liability drug rules of sports governing bodies. *New Law J 1996;***2**: 1161–1164.

5 IAAF. *International Amateur Athletic Federation handbook.* Monaco: IAAF, 2000.

6 International Olympic Committee. *Olympic movement anti-doping code.* Lausanne: IOC, 1999.

7 UK Sport. *Anti-doping programme: Annual report 1999–2000.* London: UK Sport, 2000.

8 Vieweg K. *A legal analysis of the German Situation.* Paper presented to the international symposium on doping in sport and its legal and social control, Birmingham, Alabama, 1996.

9 Tarasti L. *Legal solutions in international doping cases: Awards by the IAAF Arbitration Panel 1985–1999.* Milan: SEP Editrice, 2000.

10 Australian Sports Drug Agency. *Survey of elite athletes.* Canberra, Australia: ASDA, 1995.

11 Sports Council. *Doping control in the UK: A survey of the experiences and views of elite competitors, 1995.* London: The Sports Council, 1996.

12 De Groot S, Hartgens F, Zweers MF. *Enquete ondor topsporters over doping, doping controles en medicijn-gebruik in de sport.* Rotterdam/Arnhem: Nederlands Centrum voor Dopingvraagstukken/NOC*NSF, 1999.

13 Canadian Centre for Ethics in Sport. *National school survey on drugs and sport.* Ottawa: CCES, 1993.

14 *Cycling News*, December 1997.

15 Laure P. Doping in sport: doctors are providing drugs. *Br J Sports Med* 1997;**31**: 258–9.

16 Australian Sports Drug Agency. (1996) *Survey of National Coaches 1996*, Canberra: ASDA.

17 Council of Europe and European Union. *The Clean Sport Guide.* Brussels: 1996.

18 Australian Sports Drug Agency. *Newsletter, Vol.4.1.* Canberra: ASDA, 2000.

19 Coomber R. Effect of drug use in sport. *J of Performance Enhancing Drugs* 1996;**1**: 16–20.

20 Goode E. *Between politics and reason: The drug legalization debate.* New York: St Martin's Press, 1997.

21 Waddington, I. *Sport, health and drugs*. London and New York: E&FN Spon, 2000.
22 Korkia PK, Stimson GV. *Anabolic Steroid Use in Great Britain: an exploratory investigation*. The Centre for Research on Drugs and Health Behaviour. A report for the Department of Health, the Welsh Office and the Chief Scientist Office. Scottish Home and Health Department, 1993.
23 UK Sport. *Draft Statement of Anti-Doping Policy*. London: UK Sport, 2001.
24 UK Sport. *Statement of anti-doping policy*. London: UK Sport, 2000.
25 UK Sport. *Ethics and anti-doping: Statement of Anti-Doping Policy Fact Sheet*. London: UK Sport, 2000.
26 Council of Europe. *Anti-doping convention*. Strasbourg, 16 September 1989.

7: The role and responsibilities of doctors in doping in sport

Introduction

In recent years the General Medical Council and the World Medical Association have released statements about doctors' professional conduct in relation to doping in sport (see Chapter 2), that it is unethical and against the medical ethical codes for a doctor to provide drugs or treatment for doping.

Both doctors directly involved in sports and ordinary GPs may well be exposed to competitive sportsmen and women who have turned to drugs and doping methods to enhance their performance or physique. Club/team doctors, as well as maintaining the health of athletes, have also become increasingly involved in improving their performance. This has become a highly scientific process, often involving legitimate drugs.[1] Club/team doctors must also work in partnership with UK Sport, coaches, and national governing bodies (NGBs) to ensure the success of the anti-doping programme.

Ethical issues for general practitioners

It has been suggested that the main treatment provider for sports- and exercise-related medicine in the UK is the GP.[2] The involvement of GPs with drugs in sports may be at two levels. A patient who is taking, or thinking of taking, anabolic steroids or other drugs such as insulin for performance enhancement may ask for advice and monitoring from his or her GP. Or, a sports person may require medication for a therapeutic purpose which may or may not contravene the regulations for his or her sport. Each of these situations presents challenges for the GP that are discussed below.

The general practitioner's responsibility to the patient

In a letter to the *British Journal of Sports Medicine*[3] one GP wrote:

I am a general practitioner with a small practice but have at least two anabolic steroid users about whom I am profoundly worried. Should I ignore them, should I report them to the police, or should I give them monitoring and advice?

Finally, where do I go for the advice? One has hypertension, and a mild liver enzyme rise due to the steroids, and the other now has left sided gynaecomastasia. He tells me tamoxifen would be effective at reducing this. I believe him. Do I give it to him?

The doctor's primary duty is to act in the best interests of his or her patient. In order to do this the doctor needs all the relevant information, including information about the use of anabolic steroids or other drugs. Fostering a relationship of trust, so that patients feel confident to impart this information, is an important part of achieving that overall aim. Patient confidentiality is an essential requirement for the development of that trust and for ensuring that patients are not deterred from seeking medical attention when necessary. As with the use of other drugs, patients need to be confident that knowledge of their drug use will remain within the confidential domain of the doctor, and that the patient can talk openly about the issue without fear of recrimination or reporting. The duty of confidentiality is not absolute, however, and patients should not be given false assurances about the extent of that duty. Information may be disclosed, without consent, where there is an overriding public interest. This usually applies where failure to disclose information would leave the patient, or someone else, at risk of death or serious harm. In the absence of such an overriding public interest, however, on balance it is probably more conducive to patient health and safety that information about the use of anabolic steroids should remain confidential. Nevertheless, as with any other potentially damaging habit (such as smoking or alcohol addiction) doctors should clearly warn patients of the dangers of such abuse.

Although doctors are prohibited from prescribing, or colluding in the prescription of, anabolic steroids or other drugs for performance enhancement in sport, the GMC does not prohibit doctors from providing "any care or treatment where the doctor's intention is to protect or improve the patient's health". This allows for doctors to participate in needle exchange facilities and to offer advice and guidance about the use of anabolic steroids and other drugs in the type of harm reduction exercise referred to earlier in this report. Some people would argue that by offering such advice and monitoring the doctor is condoning and perhaps encouraging continued use of illicit drugs. Although the position may not be an entirely comfortable one for doctors, a pragmatic approach that seeks to promote the best interests of the individual patient represents the best option in a difficult situation. As mentioned above, giving advice would, of course, include providing information about the risks and dangers of using anabolic steroids and other drugs, and perhaps ways in which those risks can be reduced.

Considerations when prescribing for sportsmen and women

The use of medication in the treatment of sportsmen and women requires the careful consideration of the doctor. Doctors should familiarise themselves periodically with the IOC list of banned substances, and also ask themselves the following questions:[4]

- Does this diagnosis really require this medication? Could the condition be treated without any drugs (that is, pain control, viral infections, nausea)?
- Can the adverse drug-related problems be minimised? Is there a dosage form or use pattern to limit the potential problems (that is, topical or inhaled vs enteral or parenteral)?
- Is this drug banned by a sport's governing body?
- Will this drug pose a problem despite all reasonable precautions? Is this a risk-prone drug despite all prudent precautions (that is, lithium for bipolar disorder, androgens for osteoporosis)?
- Should this athlete compete while ill? Would it be more prudent and reasonable to hold this athlete out of competition while treatment ensues (for example a febrile athlete who might have carditis)?

Table 7.1 gives examples of drugs to avoid with athletes.

In addition to asking these questions, Henderson[4] advises that the doctor should be aware of problems that may arise because of the very nature of the sport in which the patient partakes:

- *Photosensitivity.* Many sports take place in the open air, and so awareness of drugs which may cause photosensitivity is important. Examples of drugs that can cause erythroderma include tetracycline, griseofulvin, thiazide diuretics, chlorpropamide, and chlordiazepoxide (Librium).
- *Autonomic inhibition.* When anticholinergic drugs are used, thermoregulation, appetite, blood pressure, libido, and alertness control can decrease. All atropine- and hyoscine-containing drugs are

Table 7.1 Drugs to avoid with athletes.

Drug group	Examples
Phototoxic drugs	
Antibiotics	Tetracycline, griseofulvin
NSAIDS	Piroxicam
Sedating drugs	
Analgesics	Narcotic analgesics
Muscle relaxants	All types
Antispasmodics	Atropine–hyoscine–scopolomine-containing drugs
Antihistamines	Non-selective histamine antagonists
Psychoactive drugs	
Hypnotic agents	All benzodiazepines
Behavioural modifiers	Anorectic agents; all stimulants
Thermoregulation inhibitors	
Drugs increasing endogenous heat	Any stimulants
	All sympathomimetics
Autonomic control inhibitors	All anticholinergics
Intravascular volume depletors	
Diuretics	Hydrochlorothiazide, frusemide
Xanthine derivatives	Theophylline, caffeine
Negative inotropes and chronotropes	
β-Blockers	Propanolol, atenolol, metoprolol
Calcium antagonists	Nifedipine, verapamil

Source: Henderson JM. Therapeutic drugs: What to avoid with athletes. *Clin Sport Med* 1998; **17**: 229–43. Reprinted with permission of WB Saunders Company.

in this group. Many of the antispasmodics have anticholinergic influences. Heat and cold injuries and the general inability to adjust to the stress of competition can be affected by anticholinergic drugs.

- *Volume changes.* When medications have a diuretic effect, this can result in decreases in circulating volume. Volume depletion predisposes to heat stroke and decreases glomerular filtration, leading to azotaemia. Xanthine derivatives, such as theophylline and caffeine, as well as diuretics, such as thiazides, are examples of commonly used drugs that can contract blood volume.
- *Central effects.* Sedation, problems with concentration, reaction time, balance, and coordination are associated with many drugs that either cross the blood–brain barrier or contribute to orthostasis.

- *Thermoregulatory inhibition.* Some drugs predispose athletes to heat stroke by either of two mechanisms: by increasing the endogenous heat production (levothyroxine, sympathomimetic amines), or by blunting the ability of the autonomic nervous system to respond to environmental stresses (antipsychotics and antispasmodics).

Information sources about prohibited drugs

Medical practitioners who want to be sure that they are not recommending or prescribing a banned drug to their patients have a number of options:

- Consult the British National Formulary (BNF).
- Consult the IOC website www.olympic.org.
- Search UK Sport online at www.uksport.org.uk.
- Telephone the national drugs information hotline on 020 7841 9530.
- If the doctor is still unsure, the sport's NGB can be contacted (see Appendix 3 for contact details).
- Consult the Monthly Index of Medical Specialties (MIMS) Companion that is produced twice yearly. This contains advice on sports medicine as a whole, stressing that GPs should be aware that some of their patients may participate in competitive sports; it outlines the relevant GMC and IOC rules. It also contains an A–Z of banned drugs, including exceptions to the bans, and the different names and addresses of national governing bodies.

In Australia, MIMS has introduced a symbol of a running athlete that designates appropriate prescribing for sports people.[5] A symbol adjacent to the name of a drug indicates that it can be prescribed; a bracketed symbol indicates that it has restrictions applicable to its use in sports people; its absence indicates that the drug is prohibited in sport. However, this system has been rejected in the UK because of potential difficulties arising from differences in banned drugs in different sports and the ever-changing IOC list.

General practitioners' knowledge about doping

A study of general practitioners found only 35% of GPs questioned were aware that guidelines on drugs in sport are to be found in the British National Formulary, and 12% believed that medical practitioners are allowed to prescribe anabolic steroids for non-medical reasons.[6] In one study in France,[7] one in three GPs had encountered doping in sport in the previous 12 months, and in a study of GPs and paediatricians in Texas,[8] over half reported having been asked about steroids or seeing possible steroid users in their practices in the previous five years.

In the French study, 61% of drug-using sports people questioned cited their GP as the source of their drugs.[7] Having adequate knowledge about prohibited medications and routes of administration is therefore important, as a number of doctors may prescribe prohibited drugs through ignorance of the IOC list, through inattention, or through being fooled by the athlete making the request. Inclusion of the subject of doping in sport in the undergraduate medical curriculum under "The Individual in Society" and "Personal and Professional Development" themes as part of the training received by doctors about drug abuse, may be considered an effective method of raising their awareness and knowledge of the problem.

There are longer-term training options available for sports medicine in general. In the UK, the Academy of Medical Royal Colleges acknowledged that doctors practising sport and exercise medicine must meet recognised standards, and to this end the Intercollegiate Academic Board of Sport and Exercise Medicine (IABSEM) was established. The UK Diploma Examination in Sports Medicine (run for IABSEM by the Royal College of Surgeons of Edinburgh) can be obtained by sitting its examination. The British Association of Sport and Exercise Medicine, in partnership with the National Sports Medicine Institute, runs a national programme of postgraduate courses. The programme is designed to cover the syllabus of the IABSEM diploma. In addition, a number of universities offer postgraduate diplomas and MScs in sports medicine, including Manchester Metropolitan University and the Universities of Sheffield, Glasgow, Nottingham, and London.

Ethical issues for sports doctors

Doctors who are employed by a sports organisation to look after the health of athletes represent one of a broader group of doctors who have dual obligations that can, potentially, lead to conflict. Such doctors may feel that their responsibilities towards the patient in such circumstances are vague and unspecified, whereas their duties to their employer or the body paying for their services may be more clearly defined. Sometimes doctors find that they have assimilated the norms and values of the employing body rather than acting in accordance with their professional standards. This is compounded by the absence of a framework for defining and regulating the role of sports doctors in clubs and organisations.[9] It is essential for all doctors to recognise that, despite being paid by a third party, they still retain a duty of care to the individual patient. They must also remember that they are still bound by the guidelines of the GMC and that they have a duty of confidentiality to the patient. Some have called for sports medicine to be brought under the umbrella of a regulatory body. Currently medical practitioners can join the British Association of Sport and Exercise Medicine and the National Sports Medicine Institute, although these are voluntary organisations. The European Group on Ethics[10] recommended that the EU should promote the drafting of a code of good practice in sports medicine; the sports physician must scrupulously respect the ethical principles of his/her profession, and specifically the safeguarding of the athlete's health.

Conflict of interest

A physician has a conflict of interest when competing interests or commitments compromise his or her independent judgement.[11,12] Doctors may have a conflict of responsibility when employed by a sports organisation to look after the health of the athletes. If it becomes apparent that a patient is using some form of illicit drug, must the doctor inform the governing/managing body – that is, his/her employer? The BMA's 1996 report states: "The medical advisor should always keep in mind the overriding duty to the individual performer, as an individual patient. Conflicts of duty between responsibility to the athlete patient and any governing or managing body should be recognised, identified and resolved in favour of the overriding professional duty to the patient". It is important that these issues are clearly articulated and formal agreement reached to avoid the doctor being pressured, for example to routinely disclose information to club managers without the patients' consent. A doctor should inform their athlete patients at the outset that he or she (that is, the doctor) may be approached for information by the governing/managing body.

Some doctors may hold the position of the medical director of a sport's NGB and simultaneously be a club's doctor. On occasions, drug test results are sent straight to the NGB, and the medical director may discover that a member of his or her club has tested positive.

Where, as in these circumstances, a conflict of interest is clearly fore-seeable, steps should be taken in advance to minimise that conflict. For example, the doctor may negotiate with the governing body that any test results from athletes for whom he or she has clinical responsibility will be handled by another doctor/officer at the governing body. This would not only avoid the potentially difficult situation regarding confidentiality, but would also reduce the risk of the doctor being accused of partiality in the handling of such results.

The establishment of an independent agency to deal with the results of drug tests could potentially prevent doctors from being placed in a difficult situation. As an additional precaution, medical practitioners should consult the medical defence unions prior to agreeing to become a team doctor, in order to discuss the potential conflicts of interest.[13]

Pressure from the organisation/body

There is a very real pressure on doctors from sporting management to pass their competitor patients as fit to compete. In the case of foot-ballers, this may involve injecting the joints with painkillers. This causes a conflict between maintaining the short-term health and the long-term health of the competitor patient. Athletes, and those work-ing with athletes, may care less about their long-term health; doctors must present the risks of this approach to the patient to assist him or her in reaching an informed decision. On occasions, a doctor may decide that an athlete is unfit to compete and should inform the ath-lete prior to informing any other interested parties. When coming to a decision, doctors should use their discretion, as "a doctor employed by a private organisation bears responsibility for prescribing and must be able to exercise independent clinical judgement, regardless of the policies of the clinic's management".[14] Doctors must speak out about any management rules that compromise health or safety or impose unrealistic demands on the athletes or themselves.[15] The best-practice model is where managers have minimal involvement with the direct management of injuries and where they accept the medical team's judgement.[9]

Pressure from the sportsmen or women

Doctors are also likely to be pressured by the sportsmen and women themselves to pass them fit to compete. They may be asked openly to provide a performance-enhancing drug to the athlete. Based on the BMA's standard ethical guidance,[16] our 1996 report advised that:

consent and autonomy are not the sole prerogative of patients and it is not only the patient who has rights of consent and refusal ... Doctors may refuse treatment that is 'bad for them' or for others. Dealing with a situation where a patient insists on a prescription that the doctor feels cannot be justified needs time for doctors to listen to patients' views and for them to explain their clinical understanding of the situation. Some doctors have proposed that if counselling fails to convince the patient of the undesirability of the requested treatment, the patient should be asked to sign a document accepting responsibility for insisting upon a prescription. Such a document is unlikely to carry any weight in law. Ethically, it would not justify doctors who provide such a prescription, contrary to their own judgement, at the patient's request.

Any doctor complying with such a request would also be acting contrary to GMC guidance and would be open to disciplinary action.

Harm reduction policies

There is an unmet medical need from drug users for qualified, confidential, and non-judgemental medical advice. As discussed in Chapter 4, research has suggested that anabolic steroid users would welcome medical involvement but are unable to obtain the supervision that they would like.[17] There was some concern that doctors who worked in needle exchange clinics might be penalised as a result of the GMC's notes concerning doping, but the guidance was subsequently altered to contain the caveat: "This does not preclude the provision of any care or treatment where the doctor's intention is to protect or improve the patient's health".

Some have advocated co-responsibility, that is, anyone knowingly failing to report the use of performance-enhancing drugs faces the possibility of censure in some form. This may be extremely unhelpful when it comes to doctors who are attempting to help their patients by reducing harm, and may very well bring into question the doctor–patient confidentiality. The primary duty of the doctor is to act in the best interests of his or her patient. If the patient is intending to use illicit drugs, there is clear benefit in the doctor's knowing this and being able to help to minimise the risk. This would include advising about the dangers of such action and suggesting practical ways in which the patient can reduce the risks. This can be difficult for doctors, who may be concerned that they are encouraging or condoning such activity, but, as with the use of other drugs, a pragmatic approach is needed in order to minimise dangers both to the individual's health and potentially more broadly in terms of public health. If doctors were to refuse to provide advice, or were to breach confidentiality, as a matter of routine where illicit drugs were involved, people would very quickly stop seeking medical advice where necessary.

Summary

Both general practitioners and sports doctors may be exposed to the use of drugs in sport by their patients. This presents a number of ethical considerations, and involves the doctors maintaining a difficult balance between supporting the patient while not condoning the doping behaviour, and maintaining doctor–patient confidentiality while working as team/club doctor.

References

1 Waddington I. *Sport, health and drugs: A critical sociological perspective.* London: E&FN Spon, 2000.

2 Nicholl JP, Coleman P, Williams BT. The epidemiology of sport and exercise related injury in the United Kingdom. *Br J Sports Med* 1995;4: 232–9.

3 Dean C. Performance enhancing drugs [letter; comment]. *Br J Sports Med* 1999;33: 140.

4 Henderson J M. Therapeutic drugs: What to avoid with athletes. *Clin Sport Med* 1998;17: 229–43.

5 Sando BG. Is it legal? Prescribing for the athlete. *Aust Fam Phys* 1999;28: 549–53.

6 Greenaway P, Greenaway M. General practitioner knowledge of prohibited substances in sport. *Br J Sports Med* 1997;31: 129–31.

7 Laure P. Doping in sport: Doctors are providing drugs. *Br J Sports Med* 1997;31: 258–9.

8 Salva PS, Bacon GE. Anabolic steroids: Interest among parents and non athletes. *South Med J* 1991;5: 552–6.

9 Houlihan B. *Dying to win: Doping in sport and the development of anti-doping policy.* Strasbourg: Council of Europe, 1999.

10 European Group on Ethics in Science and New Technologies. *Opinion on the ethical aspects arising from doping in sport.* Brussels: November 1999.

11 Rodwin MA. Medicines, money and morals: Physicians' conflict of interest. Oxford: Oxford University Press, 1995.

12 Polsky S. Winning medicine: Professional sports team doctors. *J Contemp Health Law Policy* 1998;14: 503–29.

13 British Medical Association. *Doctors' assistance to sports clubs and sporting events.* London: BMA, 2001.

14 British Medical Association. *Sport and exercise medicine: Policy and provision.* London: BMA, 1996.
15 Pipe A. Reviving ethics in sports: Time for physicians to act. *Phys Sports Med* 1998;**26**: 39–40.
16 British Medical Association. *Medical ethics today: Its practice and philosophy.* London: BMA, 1993.
17 Korkia PK, Stimson GV. *Anabolic steroid use in Great Britain: an exploratory investigation.* The Centre for Research on Drugs and Health Behaviour. A report for the Department of Health, the Welsh Office and the Chief Scientist Office. Scottish Home and Health Department, 1993.

8: Summary and recommendations

This BMA report has shown that doping in sport is a complex, deeply entrenched, constantly shifting problem. Far from being a recent phenomenon, it dates back to the third century BC. Nevertheless, in the 20th century it became more sophisticated, with the evolution of the modern pharmaceutical industry and the arrival of drug testing. Doping occurs among both elite and non-elite athletes, although its extent has not been evaluated accurately. In terms of non-elite sport, this report chose gymnasium users and their use of anabolic steroids (AAS) and other drugs as its example. The evidence, from GP and needle exchange surveys and interviews with AAS users, suggests that AAS use in British gymnasiums is sufficiently common for AAS to be considered a public health problem. Available indicators suggest that AAS use is not going to be a passing trend. Research into their potential adverse effects has been shown to be incomplete and inconclusive – a cause for concern, as they are one of the most popular classes of drugs used in the sporting world. Preventative strategies need to be put in place to reduce harm among those who insist on using AAS.

In elite sports, a much wider range of drugs and methods are used. The relatively few investigations into the prevalence of this use[1-3] have indicated that drugs are used in almost every sport at all levels. Almost 50% of British athletes questioned in the Sports Council survey felt that drug use was a problem in international competition in their sport (rising to 83% for track and field). The drug abusers are a heterogeneous category and vary, not only as a result of personal morality, but also as a result of the particular context within which they practise their sport. Key variables in that context include the demands and traditions of the particular sport, the domestic political and economic situation, and the degree of commercialisation that prevails within the sport. All these factors combine to increase the pressure faced by sportsmen and women and their entourages.

With regard to anti-doping policy, rather than construct a policy response around either a particular manifestation of the problem or one type of policy instrument, it is essential that policy is sensitive to the multifaceted nature of the issue and its dynamic quality. Perhaps understandably, policy emphasis has to date been placed on a limited range of mainly Olympic sports, and has tended to rely on sanctions as the primary instrument of policy implementation. Policy needs to be critically examined and reoriented beyond the individualistic law and order approach. Policy makers need to identify a broader range of policy instruments from which to construct a more tailored response to the problem of doping in sport. This must be conducted with full support at a domestic level, from the government and governing bodies, but also importantly at an international level too.

As the anti-doping policy is re-examined, contributions and advice from the medical profession will be important, particularly with regard to information included in the education programmes, and with the design of an effective rehabilitation programme for athletes who have failed drug tests. By increasing the knowledge and awareness of doping in sport among healthcare professionals with an interest in sports medicine, we can hope to raise the profile of the problem and better advise the sporting organisations in the formation and implementation of their anti-doping policies.

We have discussed the responsibilities of both GPs and sports doctors to their patients and the ethical issues that may arise. It is essential to remember that sports medicine is a legitimate and necessary specialist field of medicine. Sports doctors employed by sporting organisations must recognise that they have a duty of care to the individual patient. They are bound by the GMC's guidelines, and have a duty of confidentiality to their patient. Formal agreement must be reached between the doctor and the sporting organisation to ensure that the above points are clearly understood in order to prevent the doctor being exposed to difficult conflicts of interest.

It must also be acknowledged that GPs may encounter sports drug users. Health professionals need to be aware that drugs may have a significant effect on individuals who participate in sport and exercise, whether at a social level or in elite competition. For the management of illness, prescribers need to assess the necessity for drug treatment, the impact that drugs may have on performance, and whether the drug is banned in sport. A balance needs to be struck between the potential beneficial effects that drugs may impart in the treatment of illness and injury, and the adverse effects associated with their use. This report has provided information about drugs and doping methods used by athletes and banned by the International Olympic Committee, and outlined the potential adverse effects that may arise from their use. It has also provided information on therapeutic drugs used in the management of common illnesses that athletes may experience, their adverse effects, and implications for their use in sport.

The results of this study of the issue of doping in sports lead the BMA to make the following recommendations.

Education and information

Medical profession

1. Consideration should be given to the development of a code of practice for sports medicine which focuses on the sports doctor's responsibility to respect the ethical principles of his or her profession, and specifically the preservation of the health of the sports person.
2. Consideration should be given to the inclusion in the undergraduate medical curriculum of the subject of doping in sport, as part of any training received by doctors about drug abuse under the core curriculum themes of "The individual in society" and "Personal and professional development".
3. Training in drug misuse in sport should form part of postgraduate medical education for any doctor likely to come into contact with such drug misusers in their work, and should also be an essential element of any programme or course on sports medicine.
4. GPs, primary care staff and accident and emergency units should be made aware of available local harm reduction or outreach services for the treatment of patients who use drugs for non-medical purposes in sport.
5. Sportsmen and women should be encouraged to have long-term medical monitoring after giving up competition work, whether or not they were using drugs at certain times in their career, as intensive sport may lead to health problems.

Athletes

6. A framework for the evaluation and assessment of education and prevention programmes for athletes should be developed by UK Sport in conjunction with the World Anti-Doping Agency.
7. UK Sport should work together with the Health Development Agency to establish mandatory education and rehabilitation programmes for athletes who are suspended for doping offences.

Doctors should be involved in advising on the development and content of the rehabilitation programmes.

8. National governing bodies, sports clubs, and gymnasiums should be encouraged to provide the following information to their members as part of a national, structured approach to education:
   - Details of banned drugs and methods
   - The effects on health of doping
   - Contact details of the Anti-Doping Directorate at UK Sport
   - Details of local harm reduction clinics.

9. Those working with child athletes, particularly coaches and parents, should be aware of appropriate training levels for children, and the dangers of overtraining and doping.

The public

10. The Health Development Agency should be approached to assist in determining the most effective methods of raising awareness of doping in sport and the implications of doping among the public, particularly young people:
    - At school level
    - In amateur sports, especially where practised by children, teenagers, and young adults
    - Those intending to take up the professional practice of sport.

Policy

11. The UK and international doping policies to date have not led to a reduction in the number of sports people using drugs, and so have failed to ensure their wellbeing. The policy should be reoriented beyond its current emphasis on sanctions, to include other policy instruments, such as education, harm reduction, and rehabilitation.

12. The "strict liability" policy should be reviewed, and consideration given to the responsibilities of all members of the sports person's entourage.

13. An analysis of the policies surrounding testing methodologies is required.

14. The merits of the drug passport scheme should be evaluated and consideration given to a pilot scheme in the UK, with full implementation if it is shown to be successful.

Research

15. Further research is necessary:
    - To establish the motives for drug use, and differences between sports, gender, and age
    - To examine possible alternatives to current anti-doping policy
    - Into effective rehabilitation of sports people who have used drugs
    - To ascertain the true prevalence of anabolic androgenic steroid use
    - To confirm the adverse effects of anabolic androgenic steroids, particularly after long-term high-dose use
    - Into the health consequences of permitted sporting activities, that is, training methods and medical approaches to improve performance.

Pharmaceutical and manufacturing industries

16. Pharmaceutical companies should consider using markers to enable the detection of particular substances during an analytical test.
17. Those pharmaceutical companies manufacturing anabolic steroids should give consideration to the inclusion in their Patient Information Leaflets of a warning about the potential adverse effects of these drugs if used for non-medical purposes in sport.
18. Tighter controls over the supplies of drugs should be considered where the therapeutic use and number of manufacturers is limited, for example in the case of human growth hormone.
19. All dietary supplements should be clearly labelled to prevent sports people from inadvertently ingesting banned substances.

References

1 Australian Parliament. *Drugs in Sport: An interim report of the Senate Standing Committee on Environment, Recreation and the Arts.* Commonwealth of Australia, 1989.
2 Dubin CL. *Commission of inquiry into the use of drugs and banned practices intended to increase athletic performance.* Ottawa: Canadian Government Publishing Centre, 1990.
3 Sports Council. *Doping control in the UK: A survey of the experiences and views of elite competitors, 1995.* London: Sports Council, 1996.

Appendix 1: UK anti-doping programme

Source – UK Sport Council. *Competitors and Officials Guide to Drugs and Sport*. London: UK Sports Council, 2001.

UK Sport aims to prevent doping in sport and achieve a commitment to drug-free sport and ethical sporting practices. This is a continual challenge that the Anti-Doping Directorate meets through a three-pronged approach: prevention, deterrence, and education. All national governing bodies are required to implement effective anti-doping measures.

In practice, UK Sport is responsible for the implementation of an effective testing programme and the encouraging of comprehensive education programmes. UK Sport liaises closely with the Sports Councils in England, Northern Ireland, Scotland, and Wales, and with governing bodies of sport, to achieve a comprehensive anti-doping programme in the UK. UK Sport also contributes to the international fight against doping in sport through its involvement in various international projects.

The success of the UK's anti-doping programme is dependent upon an effective partnership between UK Sport and governing bodies' administrators, legal advisers, and medical officers, together with national coaches and, most importantly, the athletes themselves. The Independent Sampling Officers (ISOs) also play an important role in the success of the programme, ensuring that the strict and high standard of sample collection is maintained.

It is a condition of receipt of grants and services from the Sports Councils that governing bodies are required to implement an effective anti-doping policy.

Who does what?

In running the drug testing programme, UK Sport is responsible for the collection of samples, arranging their analysis at an International Olympic Committee-accredited laboratory, and reporting all test results to the appropriate governing body. The governing body must have adequate anti-doping regulations and jurisdiction to test its members before it will be accepted into the drug-testing programme.

UK Sport determines an effective level of testing for each sport in conjunction with the relevant governing body. A schedule of events and the training/preparation programme are provided by the governing body, which also prioritises the events, teams, and athletes at which testing should be targeted.

It is the governing body's responsibility to communicate results to the athletes. In the case of a positive finding or a refusal to comply with a request to provide a sample, a review panel must determine whether a doping offence has been committed. The independent disciplinary hearing investigates the circumstances and decides what, if any, sanctions are to be imposed. The decision of the disciplinary hearing may be appealed to an independent tribunal by either party.

UK Sport monitors the actions taken by governing bodies to ensure they are operating fairly and in accordance with their own rules, which is a condition of receiving grants and services from the Sports Councils.

Competition testing

Competition testing is when the athletes, from whom those to be tested are selected, are participating in a sporting event. Every sporting event should be open to the possibility of testing, although usually it is targeted at the elite, or potential elite-level, athletes. UK Sport authorises a team of Independent Sampling Officers (ISOs) to oversee the selection process, verify the collection of samples, and dispatch them to the laboratory by secure means.

Who can be tested?

Any athlete entering a competition or named as a member of a team participating in a competition that has been selected to be part of the drug-testing programme.

How are athletes selected for testing in competition?

The selection of athletes to provide a sample is determined by the rules of the governing body. The selection policy may target:

- Placing in the event
- Discipline, category, or round
- Random selection

- A set number of players from each team (usually using random selection)
- Those qualifying for national representation.

In many sports, such as athletics, swimming, and cycling, a record will not be recognised until a negative drug test has been returned by the athlete. Some sports require a negative drug test before they will recognise an area or national record.

To ensure fairness the selection draw is witnessed by representatives from UK Sport and usually the governing body. Depending on the sport, the draw may take place in several ways. For example, if the event involves a number of teams then the draw may begin with the selection of the round of competition when testing will take place. At a competition where several classes are competing, the draw may involve first classes, then places.

Out-of-competition testing

Out-of-competition testing is drug testing that can occur at any time of the year and in any location, such as at the athlete's home, place of training, or even while they are overseas. Out-of-competition testing usually takes place at little or no notice.

Who can be tested out of competition?

The governing body of the sport provides UK Sport with the contact details of athletes in an agreed eligible category (international representative, performance level, receipt of funding), for out-of-competition testing. The governing body should inform its athletes if they may be subject to out-of-competition testing and that they are required to provide their governing body with up-to-date contact details, including address, telephone numbers, place of work, and training venue(s).

Athletes eligible for out-of-competition testing are usually identified in one of two ways:

1. National squads/teams – all athletes named as part of the squads/teams identified by the governing body as being of the appropriate level may be subject to out-of-competition testing.
2. Register of eligible athletes (usually for individual sports) – a list of athletes who fall within an eligible category agreed between the

governing body and UK Sport. This should include all athletes in receipt of Lottery grants.

How are athletes selected for out-of-competition testing?

Athletes are selected for testing by a random draw of names, either from the squad list or from the register provided by the governing body. UK Sport conducts the independent draw to ensure fairness.

UK anti-doping programme – sample collection procedures

Although anti-doping regulations may vary from sport to sport, the sample collection procedures generally follow the same basic principles and are the same for in-competition and out-of-competition testing. The procedures in other countries usually follow the same basic principles.

The sample collection equipment that is used in other countries may vary. Available equipment includes Envopak, Versapak, and Bereg Kit 94, and is usually based on the same basic principles: the equipment should be clean and secure in tamper-resistant or tamper-evident packaging, prior to being opened by the athlete; the bottles and containers should have a unique identification system and be strong, to provide secure storage and transportation of the sample; lastly, it should also have a unique sealing system that is both tamper resistant and tamper evident.

The drug-testing procedures are designed to protect the integrity of the sampling process and ensure that it is a system that has athlete confidence. Although urine provision under the observation of another individual is not by its nature the most pleasant of procedures, the procedures are there to protect the athlete and the sport. The athletes should always know their rights and responsibilities under the governing bodies' rules and regulations.

If an athlete has not been tested before, the Independent Sampling Officer (ISO) will explain the procedures fully before the athlete gives the sample. However, athletes are advised to familiarise themselves with the procedures so that they are prepared in advance in the event that they are selected for a drug test.

All UK Sport ISOs carry an identification card which they will show the athlete upon notification that they have been selected for a drug test. The ISO will also have a letter authorising them to conduct the particular test. In other countries the system may vary; however, sampling officers must be able to show the athlete the authority given to them to collect a sample, for example an identification card, a letter from the authority requesting the test, etc.

Sample collection process

1. Notification that the athlete has been selected for a drug test at a competition or squad training session

In the UK, after an event or during training, the athlete will be notified in writing by a UK Sport ISO that they have been selected for a drug test using an official Sample Collection Form.

The athlete will be asked to sign the form to acknowledge that they have been advised of their rights and have received the notice. A copy of this notice is then given to the athlete.

The athlete is entitled to have a representative of their choice present throughout the drug-testing procedures, except in the toilet during the actual passing of the sample. The athlete may also choose an interpreter to accompany them to the Doping Control Station. With the approval of the ISO the athlete may, before they arrive at the Doping Control Station:

- Receive medical attention if necessary
- Attend a victory ceremony
- Compete in further events
- Warm down
- Fulfil media commitments
- Complete a current training session.

Out of competition

With out-of-competition testing the athlete may be given little or no notice and may initially be notified over the telephone (however, they will receive the written notification at the testing session). If the ISO contacts the athlete by telephone, he or she will need to meet the athlete as soon as possible to collect the sample, and certainly within 24 hours.

When the athlete is notified in person that they have been selected for a drug test, a chaperone (usually the ISO) must accompany them at all times until the sample collection procedure is complete. The athlete must stay in view of the chaperone at all times. Chaperoning is vital to ensure the integrity and validity of the sample and to exclude any suggestion of manipulation.

2. Reporting for testing at a competition or squad training session

A chaperone will accompany the athlete to the Doping Control Station waiting room, where sealed, non-alcoholic, caffeine-free drinks should be provided by the governing body responsible for the event. If the athlete decides to consume other drinks or food they do so at their own risk.

Out of competition

For out-of-competition testing, where no official Doping Control Station is available, the most suitable compromise is found to ensure both the privacy and the integrity of the procedures.

3. Selecting a collection vessel

When the athlete is ready to provide a urine sample, they will be asked to select a sealed sample collection vessel (from a selection of at least three) and go to the toilet area with the ISO. The collection vessel should be kept in sight of the ISO at all times throughout the entire collection process.

4. Providing a sample under supervision

The athlete must remove sufficient clothing so that the ISO can directly observe him or her providing the urine sample into the collection vessel. When the athlete has provided the required amount of urine (usually a minimum of 75ml) they must return directly to the Doping Control Station administration room with the ISO. Only the athlete, or someone authorised by the athlete, may handle the sample.

5. Selecting the sampling kit

The athlete will now be asked to select a sealed urine sampling kit (from a selection of at least three kits). Each kit is stored in tamper-evident packaging. The athlete will be asked to check that the security seal is intact. If there is any evidence of tampering, the athlete should select a new urine sampling kit. Next the athlete will be invited to break the security seal and remove the contents of the kit.

6. Dividing and sealing the sample

The athlete will then be asked to divide their sample between the A and B bottles and to seal the bottles tightly. The athlete will be asked to pour a minimum of 30ml into the B bottle and to seal the bottle, and then to pour the remaining sample into the A bottle and seal the bottle. A few drops of urine should be left in the collection vessel to allow the ISO to test the suitability of the sample for testing.

7. Checking the seal of the bottles

Next the athlete will be invited to check that the two bottles are tightly sealed and that there is no leakage (by inverting the bottles). The ISO also ensures that the bottles have been tightly sealed by checking the bottle tops. Some sample collection systems will require the bottles to be sealed in separate tamper-evident containers.

8. Testing the suitability of a sample for testing

The ISO will test the suitability of the sample for testing by measuring the pH and specific gravity of the sample. The pH measures the acidity/alkalinity of the sample, and specific gravity ensures that the concentration of urine is not too dilute.

This test is conducted by dipping an indicator stick into the remaining urine in the sample collection vessel and leaving it for a short time. A colour reaction will occur which is then compared to the colour chart on the bottle. The athlete can observe the colour-matching process. The closest-matched colour is the reading that is recorded on the Sample Collection Form.

All samples will be sent to the laboratory regardless of the pH and specific gravity reading. However, if the pH and/or specific gravity are outside the limits set by the International Olympic Committee or governing body, this fact will be recorded on the Sample Collection Form. To give further assurance to the integrity of the test, a further sample is required if the first sample collected is outside the acceptable range. This provides an additional quantity of urine in the case of a first dilute sample, or the opportunity for a comparative sample if the pH is outside the acceptable range. In this way the integrity of the testing procedure is maintained and claims of sample manipulation may be refuted.

Refusal to provide another sample may be considered by the governing body as a failure to comply with the request for testing and be dealt with as though the urine sample returned a positive result.

9. Recording the information

The ISO records the A and B sample numbers on the Sample Collection Form. The athlete should check that this information is correct. The athlete is then invited to declare any medications that they have taken during the past seven days. Although the athlete is under no obligation to make this declaration, it may be helpful in explaining a finding.

If the athlete has any comments about the drug test that they have just undertaken, these should be recorded in the comments section on the Sample Collection Form. These comments will be seen by UK Sport and the governing body, allowing for investigation of any concerns.

10. Certifying the information

The ISO then asks the athlete (and their representative, if present) to check all the information on the Sample Collection Form and, if satisfied that it is accurate, to sign the form. The ISO will also check and sign the form. The athlete will be given a copy of the Sample Collection Form and is now free to leave.

11. Transferring the samples to the laboratory

The sealed samples are placed in a security-sealed transit bag and are sent to an International Olympic Committee-accredited laboratory by a secure chain of custody for analysis – every step of the transfer process is documented and ensures that only those authorised to handle the samples do so.

The laboratory receives the copy of the Sample Collection Form, which only has details of the sample, sample numbers, and the medications declared by the athlete. No other information is provided that might allow the athlete to be identified. On receipt of the transit bag the laboratory staff will check for signs of tampering, as well as checking that the sample numbers on the Sample Collection Form correspond to the sample(s) enclosed.

Refusal to provide a sample

Although these procedures have been developed to ensure security and fairness in drug testing, the athlete can refuse to be tested. A refusal to provide a sample, however, may be considered by the governing body as though the urine sample gave a positive result. The athlete should record their reason for refusing to provide a sample in the comments section of the Sample Collection Form and sign this form. A copy will be given to the athlete as a record.

What if the athlete provides insufficient urine?

If the athlete does not provide sufficient urine, the partial sample will be sealed using a partial sample kit. This kit will have a unique number on it which will be recorded on the Sample Collection Form. The paperwork and the partial sample will be kept secure until the athlete is ready to provide another sample.

When the athlete is ready to provide more urine, they will be asked to select a new sample collection vessel and the sample will be provided under observation. The athlete will return to the administration area with the ISO. The first partial sample collection vessel will be obtained and the athlete should check the seal number on the partial sample kit and ensure that the seal has not been tampered with. The athlete will then be asked to break the seal on the kit and pour the contents of the bottle (the first partial sample) into the second collection vessel. If the sample is still insufficient in volume, the above sealing and recording procedures are repeated.

Once sufficient urine has been provided (usually 75ml) the remaining standard procedures should be followed.

UK anti-doping programme – results management

Test result is negative

Following the laboratory analysis of the A sample, if no prohibited substances are found a negative result will be reported to the relevant governing body or international sports federation and the B sample destroyed. The report is produced for UK Sport within 10 working days of the sample arriving at the laboratory. If required, results can be made available within 24 or 48 hours during a major competition.

Initial test result is positive

If a prohibited substance is found in the A sample, the governing body or international sports federation is notified of the finding. The governing body or international sports federation, after confirming the accuracy of the documentation and supporting evidence of a contravention of its rules, then notifies the athlete of the finding.

In the case of a finding in the A sample, the procedure is as documented in the Statement of Anti-Doping Policy:

1. The initial finding and supporting documentation are reviewed by a review panel to decide whether there is a case to answer.
2. If the governing body rules so require, the athlete may be suspended from competition. The athlete is invited to explain the presence of the prohibited substance in their urine sample. If the athlete does not agree with the A sample finding and wants to challenge the identity or integrity of the sample, they are entitled to be present or represented at the analysis of the B sample. This is the opportunity to formally confirm the identity of the sample and to verify the integrity of sealing.
3. If the B sample analysis confirms the findings in the A sample, or the athlete accepts the A sample finding, they are given an opportunity to present their case to an independent disciplinary committee. A decision will be made by the committee, which may include suspension from competition for a given period or, in some cases, a lifetime ban.
4. The athlete or governing body is entitled to appeal against the decision through an independent appeal tribunal.

Contact UK Sport

Telephone: 020 7841 9500
Address: 40 Bernard Street, London WC1N 1ST

Appendix 2: Laboratory analysis procedure

Source – International Olympic Committee. *Olympic Movement Anti-doping Code*. IOC, 28 May 2000 update.

The following techniques are used at the IOC-approved laboratories for testing samples:

- Gas chromatography
- High-pressure liquid chromatography
- Mass spectrometry in combination with gas chromatography
- High-resolution mass spectrometry or tandem mass spectrometry
- Immunoassay
- Additional or alternative techniques recommended by IOC Medical Commission according to new scientific developments.

The following procedures represent the minimum requirements for accredited laboratories of the IOC Medical Commission:

For volatile doping agents excreted free: Gas chromatography screening with a nitrogen-specific detector (nitrogen phosphorus detector, NPD) and capillary column, cross-linked with a moderate polarity phase. Alternative detection by mass spectrometry may be used.

For non-volatile doping agents excreted as conjugates: Gas chromatography/mass spectrometry screening after hydrolysis and extraction, derivatisation, cross-linked capillary column chromatography, and detection by selected ion monitoring (mass-specific detection).

For caffeine quantification: High-pressure liquid chromatography.

For anabolic steroids:

1. For free steroids: extraction, derivatisation, and detection by selected ion monitoring (mass-specific detection or nitrogen-specific detection. Complementary appropriate immunoanalytical methods may be used).

2. For free and conjugated steroids: after enzymatic hydrolysis, extraction, derivatisation, and detection by selected ion monitoring (mass-specific detection). Alternatively, separate extracts of the free and the conjugated fractions may be performed, each one treated and analysed as described above.

3. For low concentrations of anabolic agents, analytical methods capable of detecting levels of 2ng/ml, such as high-resolution mass spectrometry and tandem mass spectrometry, are required by the laboratories accredited by the IOC for doping control analyses. Validation data for other techniques should be presented to the Subcommission on Doping and Biochemistry of Sport for their approval.

For acidic substances, for example diuretics and probenecid: Extraction at suitable pH and derivatisation, gas chromatography/ mass spectrometry, with detection by full scan or selected ion monitoring (mass-specific detection). Alternatively, extraction and analysis by high-pressure liquid chromatography.

For hCG: A validated immunoassay to detect and quantify hCG. For confirmation, a second, different, immunoassay is required.

For other peptidic hormones: Specific techniques and methodologies will be needed following the evolution of scientific knowledge in this field. Refer to the IOC Medical Commission for updated information.

Appendix 3: Contact details of UK national governing bodies

National governing body	Contact details
Airsports	
Royal Aero Club of United Kingdom	Tel 0116 2531051 Fax 0116 2515939
British Gliding Association	Tel 0116 2531051 Fax 0116 2515939 Email bga@gliding.co.uk Web www.gliding.co.uk
British Hang-Gliding and Para-gliding Association	Tel 0116 2611322 Fax 0116 2611323 Email office@bhpa.co.uk Web www.bhpa.co.uk
British Microlight Aircraft Association	Tel 01869 338888 Fax 01869 337116 Email general@bmaa.org. Web www.bmaa.org
British Model Flying Association	Tel 0116 2440028 Fax 0116 2440645 Email admin@bmfa.org Web www.bmfa.org
American football	
British American Football Association	Tel 01661 843179 Fax 01661 843179 Email gmblade@aol.com Web www.gridironuk.com

Angling

Salmon and Trout Association	Tel 020 72835838
	Fax 020 76265137
	Email salmon.trout@virgin.net
	Web www.salmon-trout.org.uk

Archery

The Grand National Archery Society	Tel 01952 677888
	Fax 01952 606019
	Email enquiries@gnas.org
	Web www.gnas.org

Athletics

UK Athletics	Tel 0121 456 8708
	Fax 0121 456 8751
	Email information@ukathletics.org.uk
	Web www.ukathletics.org

Badminton

British Badminton Olympic Committee 2000 Ltd	Tel 01846 662577

Badminton Association of England	Tel 01908 268400
	Fax 01908 268412
	Email enquiries@baofe.co.uk
	Web www.baofe.co.uk

Badminton Union of Ireland	Tel 003531 839 3028
	Fax 003531 839 3028
	Email bui@iol.ie
	Web www.badmintonireland.com

Scottish Badminton Union	Tel 0141 4451218
	Fax 0141 4251218
	Email enquiries@scotbadminton.demon. co.uk
	Web www.scotbadminton.demon.

co.uk

Welsh Badminton Union	Tel 029 20222082
	Fax 029 20394282
	Email wbu@btclick.com
	Web www.welshbadminton.net

Baseball

British Baseball Federation	c/o BaseballSoftball UK
	Tel 020 74537055
	Fax 020 74537007
	Email info@baseballsoftballuk.com
	Web www.baseballsoftballuk.com

Basketball

English Basketball Association	Tel 0113 2361166
	Fax 0113 2361022
	Email enquiries@ebbaonline.net
	Web www.basketballengland.org.uk

| Ulster Basketball Association | Tel 028 90648000 |

Basketball Scotland	Tel 0131 3177260
	Fax 0131 3177489
	Email enquiries@basketball-scotland.com
	Web www.basketball-scotland.com

Basketball Association of Wales	Tel 029 20496696
	Fax 029 20496696
	Email fdaw@lifestyle.org.uk
	Web www.bballwales@enta.net

Biathlon

British Biathlon Union	Tel 01874 730562
	Fax 01874 730049
	Email info@britishbiathlon.com
	Web www.britishbiathlon.com

Bobsleigh

British Bobsleigh Association	Tel 01722 340014
	Fax 01722 340014
	Email bba@dial.pipex.com

Bowls

English Bowling Association	Tel 01903 820222
	Fax 01903 820444
	Email eba@bowlsengland.com
	Web www.bowlsengland.com

Irish Bowling Association — Tel 028 9065 5076
Fax 028 9065 5076
Email iba@btinternet.com
Web www.iba.btinternet.com

Scottish Bowling Association — Tel 0141 221 8999
Fax 0141 221 8999
Email scottishbowling@aol.com

Welsh Bowling Association — Tel 01597 823544
Fax 01691 831486
Email mike.lan@onetel.net.uk

English Women's Bowling Association — Tel 01926 430686
Fax 01926 332024
Email pabtebay@dialstart.net

Irish Women's Bowling Association — Tel 028 9268 8254
Fax 028 9268 8808

Scottish Women's Bowling Association — Tel 01475 724676
Fax 01475 724676
Email eleanor@swaba.co.uk

Welsh Women's Bowling Association — Tel 01547 528331
Fax 01547 528331
Email linda@wwba.freeserve.co.uk

Boxing

Amateur Boxing Association of England — Tel 020 87780251
Fax 020 87789324
Email hq@abae.org.uk

Welsh Amateur Boxing Association — Tel 029 20623566

Canoeing
British Canoe Union

Tel 0115 9821100
Fax 0115 9821797
Email info@bcu.org.uk
Web www.bcu.org.uk

Caving
National Caving
Association

Tel 020 84229668
Email admin@nca.org.uk
Web www.nca.org

Croquet
Croquet Association

Tel 020 77363148
Fax 020 77363148
Email caoffice@croquet.org.uk
Web www.croquet.org.uk

Crossbow
National Crossbow
Federation of
Great Britain

Tel 01932 700180
Fax 01932 700180
Email ncfgb@aol.com

Curling
English Curling
Association

Tel 01895 201000
Fax 01895 201001
Email eric@fhinds.co.uk
Web www.englishcurling.com

Royal Caledonian
Curling Club

Tel 0131 3333003
Fax 0131 3333323
Email secretaryandoffice@rccc1.
fsbusiness.co.uk
Web www.rccc.org.uk

Welsh Curling
Association

Tel 0151 6083691
Fax 0151 6083691

Cycling
British Cycling
Federation

Tel 0161 2302301
Fax 0870 871 2001
Email info@bcf.uk.com
Web www.bcf.uk.com

Disability sports

British Blind Sport	Tel 01926 424247
	Fax 01926 427775
	Email blindsport@btinternet.com
	Web www.britishblindsport.org.uk
British Deaf Sports	Tel 01943 850214
Council	Fax 01943 850828
British Wheelchair	Tel 01296 395995
Sports Foundation	Fax 01296 424171
	Email enquiries@britishwheelchairsports.org
	Web www.britishwheelchairsports.org
Cerebral Palsy Sport	Tel 0115 9401202
	Fax 0115 9402984
	Email info@cpsport.org
	Web www.cpsport.org
Disability Sport	Tel 028 90508255
Northern Ireland	Fax 028 90508256
	Email email@dsni.co.uk
	Web www.dsni.co.uk
English Federation of	Tel 0161 2475294
Disability Sport	Fax 0161 2476895
	Email federation@efds.co.uk
	Web www.efds.co.uk
Scottish Disability Sport	Tel 0131 317 1130 / 01592 415700
	Fax 0131 317 1075 / 01592 415710
	Email ssadsds@aol.com
	Web www.scottishdisabilitysport.com
United Kingdom Sports	Tel 020 73541030
Association for People	Fax 020 73542593
with Learning Disability	Email office@uksapld.freeserve.co.uk

Dragon boat racing

British Dragon Boat
Racing Association

Tel 01295 770734
Fax 01295 770734
Email dacogswell@aol.com
Web www.dragonboat.com

Equestrianism

British Equestrian
Federation

Tel 024 76698871
Fax 024 76696484
Email info@bef.co.uk
Web www.bef.co.uk

Fencing

British Fencing
Association

Tel 020 87423032
Fax 020 87423033
Email british_fencing@compuserve.com
Web www.britishfencing.com

Football

The Football Association

Tel 020 72624542
Fax 020 74020486
Web www.the-fa.org

Irish Football Association

Tel 02890 669458
Fax 02890 667620
Email enquiries@irishfa.com
Web www.irishfa.com

Scottish Football
Association

Tel 0141 616 6000
Fax 0141 616 6001
Email info@scottishfa.co.uk
Web www.scottishfa.co.uk

Football Association
of Wales

Tel 029 20372325
Fax 029 20343961
Email dcollins@faw.co.uk

Golf

English Golf Union

Tel 01526 354500
Fax 01526 354020
Email info@englishgolfunion.org
Web www.englishgolfunion.org

Scottish Golf Union	Tel 01382 549500 Fax 01382 549510 Email sgu@scottishgolf.com Web www.scottishgolf.com
Welsh Golfing Union	Tel 01633 430830 Fax 01633 430843 Email wgu@welshgolf.org
Ladies Golf Union	Tel 01334 475811 Fax 01334 472818 Email info@lgu.org.uk Web www.lgu.org.uk
English Ladies Golf Association	Tel 0121 4562088 Fax 0121 4545542 Email office@englishladiesgolf.org.uk Web www.englishladiesgolf.org
Irish Ladies Golf Union	Tel 353 1 2696244 Fax 353 1 2838670 Email info@ilgu.ie Web www.ilgu.ie
Scottish Ladies Golfing Association	Tel 01382 549502 Fax 01382 549512 Email slga@scottishgolf.com Web www.scottishgolf.com
Welsh Ladies Golf Union	Tel 01633 422911 Fax 01633 422911

Gymnastics

British Gymnastics	Tel 01952 820330 Fax 01952 820326 Email info@baga.co.uk Web www.baga.co.uk

Handball

British Handball Association	Tel 01706 229354 Fax 01706 229354 Email office@britishhandball.com Web www.britishhandball.com

Hockey

Great Britain Olympic Hockey Board	Tel 0870 1200729
English Hockey Association	Tel 01908 544652 Fax 01908 544640 Email marym@englishhockey.org Web www.hockeyonline.co.uk
Irish Hockey Association (Ulster Branch)	Tel 028 90383819 Fax 028 90682757 Email ulsterhockey@houseofsport-ni.org.uk Web www.houseofsport-ni.org.uk/ulsterhockey
Scottish Hockey Union	Tel 0131 453 9070 Fax 0131 453 9079 Email info@scottish-hockey.org.uk Web www.scottish-hockey.org.uk
Welsh Hockey Union	Tel 029 20233257 Fax 029 20233258 Email welsh.hockey@whu.softnet.co.uk Web www.welsh-hockey.co.uk

Hovering

Hovercraft Club of Great Britain	Tel 01949 837294 Fax 01949 837294 Email info@hovercraft.org.uk Web www.hovercraft.org.uk

Ice hockey

Ice Hockey UK	Tel 0115 9241441 Fax 0115 9243443 Email hockey@icehockeyuk.co.uk Web www.icehockeyuk.co.uk

Ice skating

National Ice Skating Association of UK	Tel 0115 853 3100 Fax 020 77392445 Email nisa@iceskating.org.uk Web www.iceskating.org.uk

Judo

British Judo Association

Tel 0116 2559669
Fax 0116 2559660
Email britjudo@aol.com
Web www.britishjudo.org.uk

Ju-jitsu

British Ju-Jitsu
Association

Tel 01277 224057
Fax 01277 224057
Email janetparker@bjjagb.demon.co.uk

Karate

English Karate
Governing Body

Tel 01302 337645
Fax 01302 729109
Email info@ekgb.org.uk
Web www.ekgb.org.uk

Kendo

British Kendo
Association

Tel 01788 891975
Email bka@dircon.co.uk
Web www.kendo.org.uk

Korfball

British Korfball
Association

Tel 01622 813115
Fax 01622 817148
Email bka@globalnet.co.uk
Web www.british-korfball.org.uk

Lacrosse

English Lacrosse
Association

Tel 0121 7734422
Fax 0121 7530042
Email info@englishlacrosse.co.uk
Web www.englishlacrosse.co.uk

Scottish Lacrosse
Association

Tel 01334 472126/460508
Fax 01334 476152

Welsh Lacrosse
Association

Tel 029 20708966
Fax 029 20708588
Email chrisshumack@yahoo.com

Life saving

Royal Life Saving
Society UK

Tel 01789 773994
Fax 01789 773995
Email mail@rlss.org.uk
Web www.lifesavers.org.uk

Surf Life Saving
Association of
Great Britain

Tel 01752 253911
Fax 01752 253912
Email mail@lifeguards.org.uk
Web www.lifeguards.org.uk

Luge

Great Britain Luge
Association

Tel 01684 576604
Fax 01684 891063
Web www.gbla.org.uk

Modern pentathlon

Modern Pentathlon
Association of
Great Britain

Tel 0118 9817181
Fax 0118 9816618
Email mpagb@easynet.co.uk
Web www.mpagb.org.uk

Motorcycling

Auto-Cycle Union

Tel 01788 566400
Fax 01788 573585
Email geoff.wilson@acu.org.uk
Web www.acu.org.uk

Motor sports

Royal Automobile Club
Motor Sports Association

Tel 01753 681736
Fax 01753 682938
Web www.msauk.org

Mountaineering

British Mountaineering
Council

Tel 0161 4454747
Fax 0161 4454500
Email office@thebmc.co.uk
Web www.thebmc.co.uk

Netball

All England Netball Association Ltd	Tel 01462 442344 Fax 01462 442343 Email info@aena.co.uk Web www.england-netball.co.uk
Northern Ireland Netball Association	Tel 028 90383806 Fax 028 90682747 Email netballni@houseofsport.fsnet.co.uk
Netball Scotland	Tel 0141 5704016 Fax 0141 570 4017 Email netballscotland@btinternet.com
Welsh Netball Association	Tel 029 20237048 Fax 029 20226430 Email welshnetball@mcmail.com Web www.welshnetball.org.uk

Orienteering

British Orienteering Federation	Tel 01629 734042 Fax 01629 733769 Email bof@bof.cix.co.uk Web www.britishorienteering.org.uk

Parachuting

British Parachute Association	Tel 0116 2785271 Fax 0116 2477662 Email skydive@bpa.org.uk Web www.bpa.org.uk

Polo

Hurlingham Polo Association	Tel 01367 242828 Fax 01367 242829 Email enquiries@hpa-polo.co.uk Web www.hpa-polo.co.uk

Roller hockey

National Roller Hockey Association	Tel 01462 484022 Fax 01462 484022 Email keith@rollerhockey.demon.co.uk Web www.nrha.demon.co.uk

Rugby league

The Rugby Football League	Tel 0113 2329111
	Fax 0113 2323666
	Email rfl@rfl.uk.com
	Web www.rugby-league.org

British Amateur Rugby League Association	Tel 01484 544131
	Fax 01484 544185
	Email info@barla.org.uk
	Web www.barla.org.uk

Rugby union

Rugby Football Union	Tel 020 88922000
	Fax 020 88929816
	Email rfu@rfu.com
	Web www.rfu.com

Irish Rugby Football Union (Ulster Branch)	Tel 028 90649141
	Fax 028 90491522

Scottish Rugby Union	Tel 0131 3465000
	Fax 0131 3465001
	Email rugby@sru.org.uk
	Web www.sru.org.uk

Welsh Rugby Union	Tel 029 20781700
	Fax 029 20225601

Rugby Football Union for Women	Tel 01635 42333
	Fax 01635 43016
	Email info@rfu-wanen.co.uk
	Web www.rfu-wanen.co.uk

Scottish Women's Rugby Union	Tel 0131 3465163
	Fax 0131 3465001
	Email barbra.wilson@sru.org.uk

Welsh Women's Rugby Union	Tel 029 20781737
	Fax 029 2022 5384
	Email rhodges@wru.co.uk
	Web www.wru.co.uk

Sailing

Royal Yachting
Association

Tel 023 80627400
Fax 023 80629924
Email admin@rya.org.uk
Web www.rya.org.uk

Scuba diving

British Sub-Aqua Club

Tel 0151 3506200
Fax 0151 3506215
Email webmaster@bsac.com
Web www.bsac.com

Shooting

Great Britain Target
Shooting Federation

Tel 01702 219395
Fax 01702 219250
Email km@gbtsf.freeserve.co.uk

Skiing and snowboarding

British Ski and
Snowboard Federation

Tel 0131 4457676
Fax 0131 4457722
Email britski@easynet.co.uk
Web www.complete-skier.com

British Association of
Snowsports Instructors

Tel 01479 861717
Fax 01479 861718
Email basi@basi.co.uk
Web www.basi.org.uk

Softball

British Softball
Federation

Tel 020 74537055
Fax 020 74537007
Email info@baseballsoftballuk.com
Web www.baseballsoftballuk.com

Squash

England Squash

Tel 0161 2314499
Fax 0161 2312341
Email englandsquash@squash.co.uk
Web www.englandsquash.com

Ulster Squash	Tel 028 90381222 Fax 028 90682757 Email eunicerankin@ulstersquash.fsnet.co.uk Web www.ulstersquash.co.uk
Scottish Squash	Tel 0131 3177343 Fax 0131 3177734 Email scottishsquash@aol.com Web www.scottishsquash.org
Squash Wales	Tel 01633 682108 Fax 01633 680998 Email squash.wales@tesco.net Web www.squashwales.co.uk

Surfing

British Surfing Association	Tel 01736 360250 Fax 01736 331077 Email colin@britsurf.demon.co.uk Web www.britsurf.co.uk

Swimming

Amateur Swimming Federation of Great Britain	Tel 01509 618700 Fax 01509 618701 Email cserv@asagb.org.uk Web www.britishswimming.org

Table tennis

English Table Tennis Association	Tel 01424 722525 Fax 01424 422103 Email admin@ettahq.freeserve.co.uk Web www.etta.co.uk
Ulster Branch, Irish Table Tennis Association	Tel 028 90381222 Fax 028 90682757
Scottish Table Tennis Association	Tel 0131 3178077 Fax 0131 3178224 Email ralph@stta.freeserve.co.uk Web www.tabletennisscotland.com

Table Tennis Association
of Wales

Tel 01495 756112
Fax 01495 763025
Email steve.gibbs@btinternet.com
Web www.btinternet.com/ttaw

Tae kwon-do
British Tae Kwon-Do
Council

Tel 0117 9551046
Fax 0117 9550589

Lawn tennis
Lawn Tennis Association

Tel 020 73817000
Fax 020 73815965
Web www.lta.org.uk

Tennis and rackets
Tennis and Rackets
Association

Tel 020 73863448
Fax 020 73857424
Email ceo@tennis-rackets.net

Tenpin bowling
British Tenpin Bowling
Association

Tel 020 84781745
Fax 020 85143665
Email admin@btba.org.uk
Web www.btba.org.uk

Triathlon
British Triathlon
Association

Tel 01509 228321
Fax 01509 223931
Email information@britishtriathlon.co.uk
Web www.britishtriathlon.org

Tug-of-war
Tug-of-War Association

Tel 01494 783057
Fax 01494 792040
Email info@tugofwar.co.uk
Web www.tugofwar.co.uk

Volleyball
English Volleyball
Association

Tel 0115 981 6324
Fax 0115 945 5429
Email general@eng-volleyball.demon.co.uk
Web www.volleyballengland.org

Northern Ireland Volleyball Association	Tel 028 97533734 Fax 028 97533734

Scottish Volleyball
Association

Tel 0131 5564633
Fax 0131 5574314
Email sva@callnetuk.com

Water skiing
British Water Ski
Federation

Tel 020 78332855
Fax 020 78375879
Email gill@bwsf.co.uk
Web www.britishwaterski.co.uk

Weight lifting
British Weight Lifting
Association

Tel 01865 200339
Fax 01865 790096
Email twister@clara.co.uk
Web www.bawla.com

Wrestling
British Amateur
Wrestling Association

Tel 01246 236443
Fax 0161 8331120
Web www.britishwrestling.org

Yoga
British Wheel of Yoga

Tel 01529 306851
Fax 01529 303233
Email office@bwy.org.uk
Web www.bwy.org.uk

Index

Page numbers in **bold** type refer to figures; those in *italic* refer to tables or boxed material